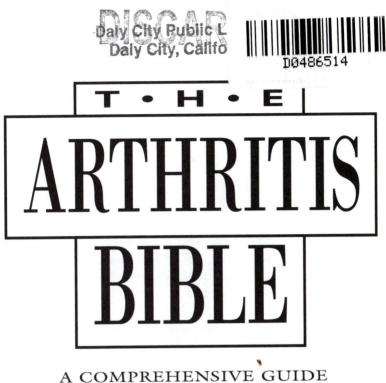

T·H·E
ARTHRITIS
BIBLE

A COMPREHENSIVE GUIDE
TO ALTERNATIVE THERAPIES AND
CONVENTIONAL TREATMENTS FOR
ARTHRITIC DISEASES

CRAIG WEATHERBY
LEONID GORDIN, M.D.

Healing Arts Press
Rochester, Vermont

S

Healing Arts Press
One Park Street
Rochester, Vermont 05767
www.InnerTraditions.com

Healing Arts Press is a division of Inner Traditions International

Note to reader: This book is intended as an informational guide. The remedies,
approaches, and techniques described herein are meant to supplement, and not to be a
substitute for, professional medical care or treatment. They should not be used to treat
a serious ailment without prior consultation with a qualified healthcare professional.

Library of Congress Cataloging-in-Publication Data
Weatherby, Craig.
The arthritis bible : a comprehensive guide to alternative
therapies and conventional treatments for arthritic diseases
including osteoarthrosis, rheumatoid arthritis, gout, fibromyalgia,
and more / Craig Weatherby and Leonid Gordin
p. cm.
Includes bibliographical references and index.
ISBN 0-89281-825-5 (alk. paper)
1. Arthritis—Popular works. 2. Arthritis—Alternative treatment.
3. Inflammation—Popular works. I. Gordin, Leonid II. Title.
RC933.W42   1999   99-18474
616.7'22—dc21   CIP

Printed and bound in the United States.

10 9 8 7 6 5 4 3 2 1

Text design and layout by Virginia L. Scott
This book was typeset in Caslon with Bodoni and Galliard as
the display typefaces.

CONTENTS

ACKNOWLEDGMENTS

I WANT FIRST AND FOREMOST TO THANK MY WIFE, Laura Inouye, for many words of encouragement and many hours of editing and extra parenting. I am also deeply indebted to old friend and medicine hunter extraordinaire Chris Kilham, whose timely invitation led me to become a health writer. Chris also suggested the book's memorable moniker, and introduced me to Paul Koether, whose support made the research and writing possible (thank you, Paul). And my agent, Anne Sellaro, deserves great credit for being such a creative, energetic advocate.

Leonid Gordin, M.D., brought a trained, critical, medical eye to *The Arthritis Bible,* and helped me understand the pain and mysteries of arthritic diseases. His dedication, intellectual integrity, and curiosity make him an exemplary physician and most congenial coauthor. I am also grateful to Les and Lorraine Marino of the Marino Center clinic in Cambridge, Massachusetts, who facilitated our authorial collaboration.

I would like especially to acknowledge the late John F. Prudden, M.D., for his time, assistance, unpretentious attitude, and kind foreword. His pioneering cartilage therapy research deserves enduring

ACKNOWLEDGMENTS

respect and recognition. And I would be remiss not to acknowledge the brave iconoclasm of Dr. Thomas McPherson Brown. His pursuit of patient benefit in the face of institutional opposition benefited thousands and spurred vital research.

Many others provided assistance, leads, or cogent comments. I would like to acknowledge Anthony Cichoke for illuminating German research on enzyme therapy, and thank Pei Pei Wishnow, Ph.D., and Zhang Zhang Zheng, M.D., for freely sharing firsthand information on Chinese use of Lei-gong-teng and herbs in general. My thanks also go to Stephen Holt, M.D., for his candid personal views on cartilage research and his fine book, *The Power of Cartilage.* Natalie Koether, Esq., and Dr. Qun Yi Zheng, of Pure World Botanicals, provided timely support and assistance, for which I am grateful.

At Healing Arts Press/ITI, I would like to thank my very able and painstaking editor, Laura Schlivek, also Jon Graham and Rowan Jacobsen, and of course, Ehud Sperling, publisher extraordinaire. Thanks all for your kind efforts on behalf of *The Arthritis Bible.*

FOREWORD

WHEN CRAIG WEATHERBY ASKED ME TO critique his manuscript for *The Arthritis Bible,* I readily agreed to do so because I believe that current medical practice very much needs to raise its eyes to a much wider view of the problems with which we deal unsatisfactorily. In his encyclopedic survey of arthritis and rheumatoid afflictions, Craig Weatherby offers open-minded practitioners and patients a wealth of relevant, readable information not found in the usual consumer guides to arthritis, and he compellingly outlines the current legal and intellectual stasis that forces physicians into excessively narrow avenues of inquiry and therapy.

In my various roles as surgeon, teacher, and medical researcher, I have had considerable experience with the biases and institutional pressures that distort medical research and practice. My early explorations into the clinical effectiveness of various dosages of bovine cartilage involved highly encouraging trials in osteoarthritis, rheumatoid conditions, acceleration of wound healing, and, some years later, experimental treatment of advanced cancer. Unhappily, my efforts in these areas were greeted at worst with skeptical indifference by the members of medical academia and at best by fear of involvement based on a decidedly nonheroic apprehension about the effect on their careers if they were to actually try to confirm my results! This astonished me, since in my naïveté, I felt certain that the publication of results I considered epochal would provide me with an army of eager co-investigators. After all, I had shown that contrary to conventional teaching, wound healing could be consistently accelerated (previously declared a biological impossibility), rheumatoid and osteoarthritis conditions significantly improved, and advanced cancers cured with unexpected frequency by therapy with bovine cartilage. The lack of any positive reaction from colleagues and institutions whose scientific objectivity and curiosity I took for granted was originally inexplicable, but I have now concluded that the primary causes for this unexpected attitude are rooted in the nature of medical training and institutions.

Weatherby sees this clearly and ably discusses the dilemma in his preface. The basic problems are twofold: first, physicians' attitudes induced by medical school and residency experiences and, second, inconsistent and illogical government regulation that strongly influences research and provider conduct. With regard to the first, the attitudes of physicians have gradually narrowed under the zealotry of regulators and the curious therapeutic rigidity of medical schools. In this way, many providers have slowly become transformed into highly skilled technicians rather than physicians. This unfortunate change occurs when a physician becomes a slavish follower of a therapeutic "cookbook" despite the compelling fact that his or her patient is growing worse. When the patient suggests that maybe they should try (insert anything about which the patient may have heard), the doctor often responds with Olympian anger and declares, "I can't believe that you would take this unproven substance!" Astonishingly, it never occurs to the physician that the therapy hitherto used on the patient has indeed been tested—*and proven not to work!* The intellectual dilemma of such posturing never occurs to the physician-technician. It is as if the doctor has learned a catechism rather than studied medicine.

And yet, on the other side, there are the "holistic and alternate" armies announcing famous victories that have never taken place and spending their time hyping fantasies rather than conducting meticulous research studies that might prove their claims are glorious realities. Unhappily, therefore, we must say, "A pox on both your houses." We say this since both groups are treating scientific questions in an emotional rather than an intellectual manner. And both thereby diminish their opportunity to be of service to those who have come to them in hope and trust.

The ultimate responsibility clearly rests with the leaders of academic and scientific medicine because they possess overwhelmingly more of what is needed to find the truth. But truth will never be found if they reject promising possibilities raised by "lesser breeds without the law." Characteristically, all momentous new developments are initially resisted by most of those working in the affected field. Neither leading institutions nor individual investigators should ever immediately condemn ideas from left field that claim unexpected efficacy. They should bring their superior resources to the assessment of a hope that gleams from any quarter. And the law should be changed so that the Food and Drug Administration does not inexcusably slow the development of promising drugs while permitting irresponsible verbal hype for the promotion of substances labeled "food supplements." The present chaotic scene is a result of this demonstrably harmful mismanagement.

I suggest that a high-level commission be constituted to recommend reasonable changes in regulations to the Congress. It should be composed of distinguished representatives of academic medicine and freestanding scientific institutions together with appropriate spokespersons for holistic and alternative medicine, nutritionists, acupuncturists, and psychologists. The greatest hope for success against disease clearly resides in those who hold leadership roles in scientific (not bureaucratic) medicine. Great care must be taken, however, to ensure that all members of the commission approach their responsibility with an intellectual openness consistent with a fair reach for promise in the observations of nonacademic medicine. They must not interpret their membership on the panel as an opportunity for self-congratulation and confirmation. On the other hand, holistic and alternative practitioners should recognize the need for rigorous scientific examination of all treatment claims. The responsibility is primarily to our patients, not to cash flow. We need to return to what was once aptly called the "priesthood of medicine."

JOHN F. PRUDDEN, M.D., MED. SC.D.
Chairman, Foundation for Cartilage
and Immunology Research

TAKE CHARGE OF YOUR HEALTH

IN MAY OF 1998, U.S. PUBLIC HEALTH AGENCIES published a sobering status report on arthritis. According to the authors, the prevalence of arthritis is likely to increase sharply, and the disease will afflict almost one in five Americans by early in the twenty-first century. At present, arthritis is the second most common cause of work disability, after heart disease, and affects forty million Americans—a figure that is expected to grow to almost sixty million by the year 2020. In the same report, the Arthritis Foundation's medical committee chairman stated that "some forms of arthritis may be cured and we may be able to prevent other forms of arthritis." Sadly, the facts do not bear out this hope.

Arthritis, especially autoimmune varieties such as rheumatoid arthritis, can be among the most difficult diseases to treat successfully. Occasionally, mainstream medicine provides substantial relief—for a minority of cases, over limited periods of time, with adverse side effects. Of course, officially sanctioned therapies are not the only credible options. The news media are full of alternative "cures," but medical consumers lack the information needed to distinguish the credible from the laughable.

MEDICAL BIASES

Much of what medical doctors know about disease comes from a few mainstream medical journals, reflecting the limited range of research performed by top drug companies, government agencies, and universities. These institutions are absolutely central and critical to the advancement of medical science, but their research priorities do not always evidence an unbiased search for the best, safest, lowest-cost remedies. Instead, they are often driven by funding priorities, academic pursuits, professional politics, and profits. As a result, medical doctors are frequently unaware of promising alternatives. And most physicians lack the time to explore beyond the boundaries of mainstream medicine. Safe therapies that can provide significant benefit to many patients may never even cross your doctor's radar screen.

THE IMPORTANCE OF "BIO-INDIVIDUALITY"

Physicians rarely give sufficient consideration to one of the central facts of medicine—that people vary widely in their responses to therapies. Individual human beings with similar symptoms and personal characteristics often respond very differently to the same treatments. This accepted medical principle is called bio-individuality, and it is often forgotten in counterproductive debates over the merits of conventional and alternative treatments. Medical authorities will refer to bio-individuality to explain away the shortcomings of synthetic drugs, but they fail to extend the same logic to inconsistencies in the performance of alternative treatments.

In the end, arguments over the superiority of approved versus unapproved treatments are beside the point. Most of the arthritis drugs that are approved by the U.S. Food and Drug Administration (FDA) work for only a minority of patients, and most produce adverse effects. Likewise, no alternative remedy will work for all patients—but most are considerably safer than FDA-approved medical drugs. The trick is to find safe treatments that work for you, regardless of their official status. The possibilities are nearly endless; our goal is to help you limit the field to a manageable selection of promising options. In addition to approved drugs, these options should include safe nutritional and natural remedies that have significant scientific backup, a documented history of traditional use, or both.

EXPERIMENTAL THERAPIES

Recent years have borne witness to a boom in research on arthritic diseases. Many of the treatments we will review are considered experimental—that is, substances that have shown promise in research involving animals or people. Unlike the drugs sold in pharmacies and prescribed by doctors, they have not been subjected to the tests the FDA requires before approving any new drug. These requirements include animal and clinical (i.e., human) studies designed to establish a drug's safety and efficacy. Medical doctors can and do prescribe promising experimental drugs, however, providing they meet one of two sets of criteria: the drug is approved by the FDA as a medicine for any health condition or is legally classified as a dietary supplement (herb, nutrient, etc.) and has a documented history of safe use, including knowledge of potential contraindications or side effects.

Experimental therapies can include vitamins, minerals, foods, herbs, or new synthetic chemicals. No seller of a drug or dietary supplement can make claims of medical efficacy (e.g., "lessens pain of arthritis") without FDA approval. To gain even the chance of FDA approval, a company has to invest an average of twelve years and $230 million in test-tube, animal, and then human studies.[1] This is an enormous risk, since the FDA will withhold approval if the experimental substance falls short in these tests of safety and efficacy.

Drug companies cannot justify such huge risks when it comes to natural substances, which cannot usually be patented. This lack of commercial exclusivity makes it almost impossible for drug companies to recoup the costs of research, development, and regulatory approval. Medical authorities often dismiss the very possibility of efficacious but unapproved alternatives, saying that word of any such remedy would be immediately trumpeted through official channels. In fact, nothing could be further from the truth. None of the alternative therapies we will review—most classified as dietary supplements—currently enjoy FDA approval to be advertised as effective remedies for arthritis. But this says nothing about their safety or efficacy. In fact, some of these remedies are government-sanctioned arthritis drugs in Europe or Asia.

Given the demands on doctors' time, you cannot expect yours to research all the alternatives. If standard treatments work for you without undue side effects, there may be no compelling reason to explore further. But when speaking among themselves, medical experts freely admit that standard arthritis drugs fail more often than they succeed. The fact that a therapy is classified as "approved" or "unapproved" says surprisingly little about its merits and defects. It would make life easier for patients in search of relief, but the truth is more complicated than that.

If the approved remedies fall short for you and your doctor is unwilling to help you explore alternative therapies, don't go it alone. Find another doctor who is willing to serve as an open-minded guide and medical guardian. This volume is intended to provide information useful in a journey toward better health—take charge of yours. You have everything to gain and nothing to lose but pain.

WHAT IS ARTHRITIS?

ONE IN SIX ADULT AMERICANS—some forty million in all—suffers from some type of arthritis, yet it remains a poorly understood disease. The confusion is understandable, because "arthritis" is a generic term that covers several diseases affecting the connective tissues in joints, skin, and various internal organs. The term arthritis comes from the Greek words *arthro* ("joint") and *itis* ("inflammation"). But some inflammatory diseases that are lumped under the heading "arthritis" do not significantly affect the joints, and inflammation is not a primary symptom of osteoarthritis, the most common type of arthritis. Doctors now refer to this degenerative disease by the more accurate term osteoarthrosis, which means "bone–joint disorder."

To muddy the waters even more, arthritic diseases are also referred to as rheumatism, from the archaic Greek word *rheuma*, meaning "to flow." This is because most arthritic diseases (except osteoarthrosis) feature periodic inflammations and fluid buildup in and around joints or organs. Arthritic diseases fall into one of two distinct categories of disorders, each characterized by a very different set of causes and symptoms.

Osteoarthrosis (osteoarthritis) is characterized by degeneration of cartilage in joints. It may be caused by injuries, repetitive joint stress, or genetic flaws—any of which can produce imbalances in the chemical processes that maintain healthy cartilage. Osteoarthrosis is also caused secondarily by some rheumatic diseases—especially rheumatoid arthritis and ankylosing spondylitis. **Rheumatic diseases** feature inflammations resulting from immune attacks on the patient's own connective tissues, including joints, lungs, eyes, heart, and skin. Examples include rheumatoid arthritis, ankylosing spondylitis, and systemic lupus erythematosus (lupus or SLE). The one thing that all arthritic disorders have in common is a focus on connective tissue.

CONNECTIVE TISSUES AFFECTED BY ARTHRITIS

The body uses connective tissue—including cartilage, tendons and ligaments, skin, and similar tissues—to hold bones, muscles, lungs, organs, and other tissues in place. Connective tissues form and connect very small structures, such as the saclike bursa surrounding tendons and ligaments. A slippery fluid called hyaluronic acid, found in the synovial space between bones, is also important in maintaining the health of joints.

To differentiate among arthritic diseases, it is helpful to know more about the key connective tissues affected by arthritis.

Bone is very hard except in the thin, slightly softer subchondral layer at the articular (joint) ends, directly underneath cartilage. Bone constantly undergoes a process of renewal via the action of cells called osteoblasts, which build new bone, and osteoclasts, which absorb old bone.

Cartilage is a semiporous, variably elastic tissue that contains no blood vessels or nerves. Instead, cartilage is maintained by special cells called chondrocytes, which absorb old tissue and produce collagen and proteoglycans with which to build new cartilage (discussed in Chapter 4). When joints move, they automatically pump fluid in and out, simultaneously feeding chondrocytes with nutrients and removing their wastes. In addition to playing a key role in the joints, cartilage makes up the firm, nonbony structures in the nose, ears, and elsewhere.

Articular cartilage cushions the joint ends of most bones—except vertebrae in the spine—and provides a smooth surface for bones to glide past each other, almost friction free. Articular (i.e., joint) cartilage generally consists of four layers, containing varying percentages of collagen, proteoglycans, chondrocytes, and water. In fact, articular cartilage is two-thirds or more water, which it exudes under pressure and then reabsorbs. This gives it great inherent elasticity and strength, permitting surprisingly thin layers of cartilage to withstand enormous pressures on the joint ends of bones. Absent injury or metabolic upsets, the cartilage in joints can last indefinitely.

Collagen is the chief building material of skin, cartilage, tendons, and ligaments. The body can arrange this insoluble, fibrous protein in various structural patterns, each of which provides the specific combination of strength, smoothness, porosity, and elasticity appropriate to the anatomical job at hand. **Elastin** is a similar fibrous protein that helps give cartilage its amazing resiliency.

Proteoglycans are huge molecules made up of hundreds of sugar-protein-sulfur compounds called glycosaminoglycans, or mucopolysaccharides. Proteoglycans are key constituents of cartilage and most other connective tissues. As we will see in Chapters 3 and 4, their role in cartilage formation is the basis of a novel dietary therapy for osteoarthritis.

JOINT STRUCTURE

Let us start with a picture of the typical synovial joint—the type commonly affected by most arthritic diseases. You will be better able to understand your disease and prevent further damage if you can picture the way joints are put together. Synovial joints (Fig. 1) consist of five parts: a tough, fibrous **joint capsule** to hold the bones together and protect the **synovial membrane,** which secretes and encloses the **synovial fluid** in the **joint space** between **articular (joint) cartilage.** Synovial fluid serves to lubricate joint cartilage and maintain some space between the bones that form a joint.

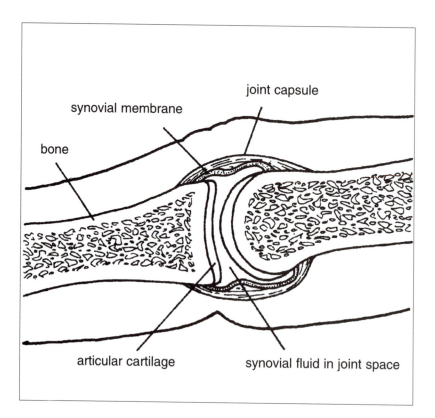

Fig. 1. Normal finger joint.

KEY SUPPORTING STRUCTURES

Ligaments, tendons, and bursa play important supporting roles in maintaining the strength and stability of joints. **Ligaments** are tough bands of connective tissue that attach bone to bone near joints. Like the joint capsule, ligaments help hold joints together. **Tendons** attach muscle to bone near joints. **Bursa** are the small, fluid-filled sacs between tendons and bone. (The term "bursitis" describes a painful inflammation in the bursa.) Now that you have a clear picture of the basic elements of joints and connective tissue, we can begin to explore the arthritic diseases and promising new options for treating them.

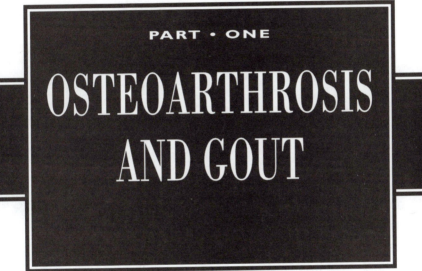

PART • ONE

OSTEOARTHROSIS AND GOUT

CHAPTER I

OSTEOARTHROSIS

(OSTEOARTHRITIS)

A CASE OF DYSFUNCTIONAL CARTILAGE

OSTEOARTHROSIS IS BY FAR THE MOST COMMON arthritic disease, with some sixteen million people seeking treatment every year and many more suffering in silence.[1] The U.S. Centers for Disease Control estimates that one in five adults will experience symptoms of osteoarthrosis by the year 2020. The term *osteoarthritis* (the old name for this condition) is more than a little misleading. As we have seen, the Greek suffix *itis* means "inflammation." But inflammation is a key symptom of rheumatoid arthritis and related diseases—not of osteoarthrosis. The new medical term, *osteoarthrosis,* means "bone–joint disorder." This new term better reflects the nature of the disease, whose primary cause of pain is the gradual decay of cartilage and subchondral bone—not the inflammation associated with rheumatic diseases (see Chapter 6).

Osteoarthrosis is not life threatening, but it can be quite disabling if left untreated. In severe cases, joint replacement surgery may become necessary. As we'll see, however, many people with osteoarthrosis may be able to avoid surgery and chronic pain with the help of physical therapies (see Chapter 2) and breakthrough nutritional treatments (see Chapter 4).

DEFINING THE DISEASE

The term osteoarthrosis describes the typical progression of events that occurs in joints affected by any of five factors, which include normal aging, physical injury, chronic joint stress, oxidative stress (free radicals from subchondral immune cells), and genetic defects. It is helpful to understand and visualize what is going on inside a joint afflicted by osteoarthrosis. Often, the first event is some sort of injury or malfunction in articular cartilage and subchondral bone. But these events may be precipitated by problems in the synovial membrane or fluid or in peripheral joint tissues—the bursa, tendons, or ligaments.

Joints are marvelous biomechanical systems whose health is maintained by a sophisticated chemical feedback loop. Problems in any part of the joint can produce a domino effect that throws the whole system out of kilter. As we age, this remarkably resilient system loses its ability to absorb stresses it handles easily at earlier stages in life. Once the system is thrown out of balance, several problems may result.

- Cartilage will roughen, fray, develop ulcers, and allow joint fluid to leak into subchondral bone, causing cysts to form in the marrow.
- Subchondral bone (that is, bone to which cartilage is attached) may develop tiny fractures, sprout jagged spurs, form calluses, and harden.
- Synovial cells may begin to form tiny pellets of bone and connective tissue called osteophytes. These collect in synovial fluid and peripheral areas of the joint, causing further damage.
- Synovial membranes thicken, reducing the joint space.

- In later stages, inflammation occurs in the synovial membrane, causing cartilage cells (chondrocytes) to manufacture the wrong kind of collagen (Types I and III, instead of the normal Type II).

This troubling picture reflects a finely tuned biochemical system that has spun out of control.

Weight-bearing joints are the ones most susceptible to osteoarthrosis, which often crops up in knees and hips as well as spinal joints. The major exceptions to this rule are ankle joints, which are rarely affected, and finger joints, which, even though they are not weight bearing, are commonly afflicted. It is also unusual to find osteoarthrosis in elbows, shoulders, or wrists.

PRIMARY OSTEOARTHROSIS

When the cause of damage is unknown—and clearly not a side effect of rheumatoid arthritis—the condition is called "primary osteoarthrosis." Throughout this book, we will follow standard practice and use the terms primary osteoarthrosis and osteoarthrosis interchangeably.

SECONDARY OSTEOARTHROSIS

When joint damage results from an injury, infection, gout (see Chapter 5), or rheumatic disease (see Chapter 6), the term secondary osteoarthrosis is used. The symptoms of secondary osteoarthrosis are often similar to those of primary osteoarthrosis, and blood tests are often needed to confirm the diagnosis.

SYMPTOMS OF OSTEOARTHROSIS

While almost everyone experiences some joint degeneration by middle age, symptoms rarely occur that soon. Because osteoarthrosis is a gradual degenerative condition, it may progress for years before making its presence felt. Nine out of ten people more than 40 years of age show early signs of osteoarthrosis on X rays but it may be a decade or more before any discomfort is felt.

The joint pain and stiffness caused by osteoarthrosis often starts as a minor annoyance. Typically, the first symptom is morning stiffness in one or more joints, which fades in a half hour or less. Stress on affected joints can cause pain, and range of motion may become diminished. Affected joints can stiffen into a bent position, feel tender, and become difficult to fully flex without pain. In some cases, including secondary osteoarthrosis caused by gout or rheumatoid arthritis, symptoms may flare suddenly and then recede for a time.

Later, arthritic joint(s) may begin to grate, crackle, and vibrate because degenerated cartilage no longer smooths the passage of bone over bone. Bony, pelletlike osteophytes may begin to block the motion of the joint. Fluid may build up, and the joint begins to swell and distort. These distortions start to stretch anchoring ligaments, causing the joint to loosen, destabilize, and produce pain. If pain discourages movement of the joint, muscles will begin to atrophy from lack of use, further destabilizing the joint.

DIAGNOSIS OF OSTEOARTHROSIS

While early signs may appear on X rays, a diagnosis of osteoarthrosis begins with the presence of symptoms perceptible to the patient. At that time, the doctor's chief concern is to differentiate primary osteoarthrosis from serious rheumatic diseases. Lab tests are useful in narrowing the diagnosis to primary osteoarthrosis (see Chapter 6).

SURGICAL OPTIONS

Should the various physical and pharmaceutical therapies described in later chapters fail to prevent crippling damage, there are surgical options. While none of these procedures is risk free or guaranteed to provide permanent relief, skilled surgery often restores disabled joints to nearly normal functioning for many years.

Arthroplasty, or **joint replacement surgery**, involves replacement of an injured joint component or whole joint with a man-made substitute. Most operations involve the hip or knee, but arthroplasty can also be performed on joints in the elbows, wrists, fingers, ankles, toes, shoulders, and jaw. **Arthroscopy** employs a long, thin tool (arthroscope) with fiber-optic capacity to examine the inside of a joint and remove bony fragments. **Osteoplasty** is the replacement of lost bone tissue, reconstruction of defective bony parts, and removal of bony fragments. **Osteotomy** is designed to alter the way bones fit in the joint by removing or adding wedges of bone. **Arthrodesis** immobilizes a joint so that the bones will grow together. This last-resort procedure prevents movement and attendant pain by permanently fusing the joint.

WHAT CAUSES OSTEOARTHROSIS?

Some cases of osteoarthrosis are believed to be initiated by injuries to joints, but any upset in the chemical system that maintains articular cartilage and bone can start a downward spiral of joint degradation and deformity. The disruption may begin with a bone defect, traumatic injury, nerve disorder, repetitive motion injury, or genetic defect. In most cases of osteoarthrosis, no precise cause can be determined. The body can usually repair minor insults to healthy cartilage, but this capacity can be foiled by genetic flaws and significant injury to or chronic stress on joints.

GENETIC FACTORS

In younger people (40 to 60 years old), osteoarthrosis often occurs in the absence of any significant injury or chronic stress to the affected joint. Many scientists have suspected that genetics is responsible for some of these "premature" cases. The genetic theory gained more support in 1996 with the publication of two reports from Britain. The first study revealed that when one of two identical twins was diagnosed with osteoarthrosis, the other was significantly more likely than the general population to have it as well. The second study found that the tissue changes typical of osteoarthrosis were more similar in identical twins than fraternal twins. (Identical twins possess the same set of genes, while fraternal twins have about half in common.)[2]

If the hereditary hypothesis is confirmed, doctors may then be able to identify the responsible genetic trait. This could allow appropriate treatment to begin before serious damage to cartilage takes place. In Chapter 4, we will review the problems these genetic traits may cause and novel dietary supplements that can limit pain by partly restoring the resiliency of cartilage.

OXIDATIVE STRESS

There is another hypothesis—excess oxidative stress—that would explain why antioxidant supplements can produce improvement in osteoarthrosis. How could oxidative stress be a factor in accelerating and worsening osteoarthrosis? You will recall that cartilage contains no blood vessels and that chondrocytes (cartilage-building cells) rely on nutrients supplied from blood vessels in subchondral bone. Changes in cartilage produced by any cause—aging, genetics, inactivity, chronic stress on cartilage, or injury—tend to reduce the blood and oxygen supply. And, ironically, cells are at greatest risk of oxidative damage when their supply of oxygen is insufficient.[3] This would help explain why antioxidant supplements produce documented benefits in osteoarthrosis—a condition that is not traditionally linked to oxidative stress.

WHO IS MOST AT RISK?

Rates of osteoarthrosis are about equal in men and women, but men tend to show symptoms earlier. Hereditary traits can cause osteoarthrosis to crop up in multiple joints or produce unique symptoms, but they are relatively uncommon. Physical activities that place repeated stress on particular joints sharply raise the risk of osteoarthrosis. Risky activities include constant kneeling, lifting, typing, and bending or a regular practice of walking or jogging on hard roads or interior surfaces in poorly cushioned shoes. "Carpenter's knee" is a perfect example of osteoarthrosis caused by repetitive stress.

Nevertheless, concern about osteoarthrosis developing as the result of a regular running routine may be unwarranted. The available evidence suggests that dedicated runners are not more likely to get osteoarthrosis in their hips or knees. As insurance, wear running shoes with ample support and cushioning and try to run on an athletic track or some other reasonably level, yielding surface—not on pavement.

Obesity was recently confirmed as a leading risk factor for osteoarthrosis in the knees. In a two-year study of women with osteoarthrosis in one knee, researchers found that those who were not obese or who lost ten pounds or more were significantly less likely to show signs of osteoarthrosis in the second knee. Participants who saw the greatest reduction in risk were the heaviest women who achieved the greatest weight loss.[4]

CHAPTER 2

PHYSICAL AND MENTAL THERAPIES

WORKING MIND AND BODY TO REDUCE DRUG DEPENDENCY

PILLS AND POTIONS ARE NOT EVERYTHING—your own actions and attitudes can have dramatic impacts on symptoms and can even affect the course of your disease. Physical therapy can be highly effective in improving strength and energy while also minimizing pain. Psychological therapies and techniques can alleviate pain and enhance the performance of your immune system. Let us take a look at the available options.

EXERCISE, PHYSICAL THERAPIES, AND ACUPUNCTURE

The pain of arthritis has an insidious side effect. People suffering pain in a joint naturally want to avoid using it. When they do, the muscles and connective tissues surrounding and supporting the joint wither, contract, and weaken. Disuse causes the joint to become progressively unstable and deformed, causing more pain. This vicious cycle can end in serious incapacitation and can dim prospects for successful joint replacement surgery. In addition, incapacitation of a knee or hip joint can keep you from getting the sort of exercise necessary for good health, immunity, and vitality.

Exercise and various physical therapies have three purposes: to maintain the flexibility, stability, and strength of joint support structures; to promote overall health; and to prevent obesity or undue weight loss. Because effective physical therapy must be customized to individual circumstances, we will outline the various types from which arthritis patients can benefit.

Your doctor may have good referrals for you, and Appendix A has tips for finding competent therapists. To help gauge the efficacy and progress of any therapy, ask for a prognosis and an estimated time frame.

CONVENTIONAL PHYSICAL THERAPIES

Exercise can help maintain the normal range of motion in joints and enhance overall strength and endurance. Joint-stabilizing exercises are of proven benefit in osteoarthrosis. One study showed a significant alleviation of pain and improvement in movement after eighteen months of targeted exercise, three times a week. The participants were older adults with osteoarthrosis of the knee who either walked or engaged in "resistance" training with dumbbells and weighted leg cuffs to strengthen muscles.[1]

Exercise can also help with rheumatic diseases, but the evidence suggests that supervised strength training improves symptoms more effectively than at-home aerobic workouts. A recent study at Tufts University indicated that rheumatoid arthritis patients who participated in a supervised program of strength training could lessen joint pain and fatigue and walk more easily. (Participating patients practiced a guided forty-five-minute strength-building regimen twice a week for three months.)[2] A contemporaneous British study produced no evidence that an at-home aerobic exercise program affected levels of fitness and fatigue in patients with lupus or rheumatoid arthritis, even after six months.[3]

Because each patient's circumstances differ, it is wise to seek professional guidance rather than rely solely on books to devise an exercise program. That said, there is a very good book called *Arthritis: What Exercises Work*, by Dava Sobel and Arthur C. Klein, which you can use as a guide and resource. In addition, the Arthritis Foundation has developed a widely praised exercise program called People with Arthritis Can Exercise, or PACE (see Appendix A).

Physical therapy can improve physical functioning and limit pain by strengthening and stabilizing joints. Most licensed physical therapists are well equipped to evaluate your condition and prescribe a customized schedule of exercises, treatments, and changes to daily routines. Physical therapists design exercise programs to help patients achieve effective relief and minimize future decline in joint health. Water provides cushioning and support that decreases stress on damaged joints, so they often suggest aquatic exercises to be performed in a pool.

Physical therapists also help by showing you how to perform routine tasks at home and work so as to minimize damage and maximize freedom of movement. They can also provide temporary relief via various treatments, including hot and cold packs, hot waxes, diathermy (electrical stimulation), whirlpool baths, and ultrasound to produce deep heat.

Physiatrists are medical doctors who specialize in musculoskeletal rehabilitation. They can design a tailored program of exercises to strengthen joints and know how to alleviate neuromuscular pain in tense, painful, ischemic (oxygen-deprived) muscles.

Occupational therapists can show you how to adjust your approach to tasks and how to use tools and movement aids called "assistive devices" to ease stress on joints. Most can also design and construct assistive devices to fit special circumstances.

MASSAGE/BODY WORK

The "laying on of hands" can help relieve musculoskeletal pain and emotional stress. With any form of massage or body work, success depends largely on the training, skill, and experience of the practitioner. If you do not feel improvement, try another technique or practitioner. Word of mouth is often the best guide to a good "body worker." Do not hesitate to ask about someone's training and experience and for client references before your first visit. You do not want to be someone's training dummy!

Massage can lift spirits and ease tense, painful muscles. Look for a state-licensed massage therapist, since unschooled amateurs can do harm. Insurance and managed care plans may pay for massage when recommended by your physician.

Neuromuscular therapy (NMT) is a school of therapeutic massage based on accepted principles of physiology and neurology. NMT practitioners apply precisely focused, calibrated pressure to improve circulation, flush out toxins, and ease tense muscles that may be pulling joints out of position. Like physical therapists, competent NMT practitioners should possess a thorough knowledge of human anatomy and be able to recommend therapeutic exercises.

Rolfing is another form of muscular therapy, similar to NMT in that it is designed to normalize posture and joint function by relaxing muscles that are tight and contracted. Rolfing differs from NMT in that it focuses on loosening muscles and connective tissues that have adhered to bone structures.

Shiatsu is an ancient Japanese massage technique. As in NMT, shiatsu practitioners apply focused finger pressure to ease pain and stiffness. Shiatsu is based on the Chinese belief that the nervous system has a bioenergetic counterpart in the form of a network of "meridians." It is said that these pathways can be stimulated with fingers (shiatsu) or thin needles (acupuncture) in ways that direct therapeutic energy to ailing tissues and organs.

Feldenkrais practitioners teach people how to walk, sit, and work in ways that help restore good posture and balance.

Yoga is an ancient Indian system of stretching, strengthening, and breathing exercises that can help improve range of motion and strengthens muscles around joints. Recently, seventeen people with osteoarthrosis in the hands participated in a clinical trial to test its benefits. They performed a yoga routine specially designed to benefit and protect the affected hands and overall body posture. Compared with eight control patients who did no yoga, those practicing the yoga routine ended the experiment with less pain and greater range of motion in afflicted joints.[4]

As the hundreds of millions of people who've practiced it over several millennia would attest, yoga also helps relieve emotional stress. The same is undoubtedly true of tai chi chuan and other ancient body–mind disciplines that emphasize flexibility, balance, and a meditative state of mind.

CHIROPRACTIC

Because of its position as the most popular alternative medical practice, this treatment deserves special mention. Chiropractic is characterized by manipulation of bones and joints, but it often includes counseling in therapeutic use of foods, supplements, herbs, and exercise. As with acupuncture, the value of chiropractic therapy depends a great deal on the training, knowledge, and skill of the practitioner. A good chiropractor will prescribe exercises to help correct musculoskeletal problems and, as needed, will refer arthritic patients for the various forms of physical therapy described here.

ACUPUNCTURE

The United Nations' World Health Organization lists acupuncture as an effective therapy for pain in shoulder and knee joints. Success with acupuncture treatment, however, depends a great deal on the training, experience, and skills of the practitioner. In one survey of arthritis sufferers, those who received treatment from trained, full-time acupuncturists fared much better than those who went to clinicians who practiced acupuncture as a sideline.

Few clinical studies on the use of acupuncture for arthritis have been conducted in the West or translated from the Chinese. The handful accessible in English show conflicting results. Some found positive effects on the immune systems of rheumatoid arthritis patients and on symptoms of osteoarthrosis and rheumatoid arthritis. Others, including one testing classic acupuncture versus "sham" acupuncture (i.e., needles inserted in the wrong places), showed little or no reduction in joint pain.[5-8] These results should be taken with a very large grain of salt, since the benefits of acupuncture depend a great deal on the training and skill of the practitioner. Performed by a competent practitioner, acupuncture is very safe and relaxing. Appendix A lists respected acupuncture schools that may be able to refer you to licensed graduates.

PSYCHOLOGICAL THERAPIES

In 1981, an experiment at the Stanford University Arthritis Center proved the value of a positive, take-charge attitude toward arthritis pain. Stanford researchers studied the effects of the Arthritis Self-Management Program (ASMP), which teaches patients about their disease and about treatments and behaviors that could have a positive impact on symptoms. The Stanford team studied three hundred patients who participated in the six-week ASMP course and a similar group that did not. On average, the ASMP "graduates" were able to cut the number of annual doctor's office visits by almost half in the first year. Four years later, the ASMP grads still reported 20% less pain and 40% fewer visits to doctors' offices. The most interesting and significant aspect of the study was the failure to find any connection between pain reduction and specific actions taken by ASMP grads. Instead, most of the benefit was derived from attitudinal changes stimulated by the ASMP training.

Most psychologists have de-emphasized Freudian-style psychotherapy for anxiety and depression in favor of cognitive therapy. Depression and anxiety are common by-products of chronic pain, and cognitive therapy has proved to be highly effective in producing rapid, positive changes. In addition, such autogenic, or "self-changing," techniques as biofeedback, self-hypnosis, meditation, guided imagery, and progressive muscle relaxation can be very helpful in alleviating stress, anxiety, and muscle tension. (These are described later in this chapter and in the interview with Dr. Leonid Gordin, which follows Chapter 6.)

COGNITIVE/BEHAVIORAL THERAPY

Mind and body are very closely connected, and for this reason cognitive behavioral therapy (CBT) employs two basic strategies to produce significant improvement in stress, anxiety, and pain. Patients are taught to adjust their behavior to minimize physical stress and fatigue, and they are trained to ignore negative thoughts and emphasize positive ones. At first, many patients dismiss the idea that "positive thinking" can limit pain, but research has proved it to be amazingly effective. Several studies at Duke University and elsewhere have found that CBT works very well, especially when spouses or others emotionally close to patients accompany them to therapy sessions. Many physicians and mental health professionals trained in pain management can help patients with CBT (see Appendix A).

GUIDED IMAGERY

If you visualize pain going away or the body healing, will it happen? Results of 1993 research at Washington State University and elsewhere suggest that this technique, called "guided imagery," works very well indeed. The Washington State team started by identifying which among sixty-five student volunteers could be easily placed in a hypnotic state. The volunteers were then divided into three groups, whose members were chosen at random.

Using group hypnotic techniques, a psychologist guided one group in visualizing that the white blood cells of their immune systems were attacking germs. They were asked to visualize this same scene twice a day, for one week. A second group floated in a tank of warm water, once at the beginning and once at the end of the week. The third control group did nothing unusual.

At the end of the week-long experiment, the students who practiced guided imagery of white blood cells on the attack showed the greatest increase in certain types of white blood cells. The students who had earlier been identified as easily hypnotized were found to have the greatest increases in white blood cell counts.

RELAXATION TECHNIQUES

Relaxation lessens stress, and less stress usually means less pain. Self-hypnosis, biofeedback, and related therapies can be highly effective in inducing physical and mental relaxation. After practicing these techniques for a while, you should be able to enter a more relaxed state at will. Many hospitals, clinics, and psychologists now offer training in relaxation techniques.

CHAPTER 3

ASPIRIN AND ITS OFFSPRING

WHILE IT MAY NOT SEEM SO TO ARTHRITIS sufferers, pain and inflammation play valuable roles in human health. Pain signals injuries that must be attended to and protected. Inflammation increases the supply of blood and immune cells to infected or injured tissues. Characterized by redness, heat, pain, swelling, and stiffness, inflammation also discourages use of the affected area.

Arthritis pain has been a primary motivation behind the ancient search for safe, effective analgesics (pain-relieving drugs). Modern analgesics can be remarkably effective in relieving pain, but many of these synthetic drugs do more harm than good. Before examining painkillers, it is helpful to understand the sources of pain in arthritis.

MECHANICAL PAIN VERSUS INFLAMMATORY PAIN

Osteoarthrosis is characterized by sharp, "mechanical" pain in or near joints, which results from loss of subchondral bone and cushioning cartilage and the resulting friction of bone grating against bone. Osteoarthrosis, however, can also produce a secondary, more diffuse "inflammatory pain" should unstable joints impinge on surrounding nerves and soft tissues. Such inflammatory pain may accompany osteoarthrosis when patients move in abnormal ways to avoid pain in damaged joints, causing formation of so-called trigger zones. (Trigger zones are areas of "referred" pain distant from the area of injury. When stimulated, trigger zones may produce pain in the injured area.)

In contrast, inflammatory pain is the main type experienced in rheumatic diseases such as rheumatoid arthritis, lupus, and ankylosing spondylitis. Inflammatory pain in the rheumatic diseases results primarily from autoimmune attacks on joint or other connective tissues. Over time, these self-destructive assaults by the immune system's white blood cells may also cause enough damage to joint tissues to produce the mechanical pain characteristic of osteoarthrosis.

ANALGESIC OPTIONS

Each year, some eighty million Americans take nonprescription synthetic analgesics, including aspirin and low-dose ibuprofen, and doctors write seventy-five million prescriptions for stronger doses or stronger drugs. Several of the most popular analgesics belong to a category of synthetic medicines called nonsteroidal anti-inflammatory drugs, or NSAIDs. The term NSAID (pronounced *en*-sed) was created to differentiate these drugs from potent steroids, such as cortisone and prednisone, which are reserved for the most painful and damaging inflammations.

Thanks to their efficacy in relieving mechanical and inflammatory pain—and the massive marketing muscle of major drug companies—synthetic NSAIDs have become the most widely used nonprescription and prescription analgesics in the world. But NSAIDs also produce dangerous side effects that kill thousands and injure many more each year. Fortunately, there are safer, comparably efficacious natural alternatives. Their advantages are explained later in this chapter (see "Safer New NSAIDs" in this chapter), and we will review each of the alternatives in Chapters 4, 12, and 13. A safer synthetic NSAID would need to mimic the action of plant-derived natural alternatives. One such synthetic NSAID currently awaits study and approval in the United States (see "Safer New NSAIDs" in this chapter).

Sometimes arthritic pain can be too severe for NSAIDs, acetaminophen (e.g., Tylenol), or the natural alternatives. Should you experience this problem, your doctor can inject the affected area with cortisone or nerve-blocking drugs or prescribe an antidepressant, narcotic, muscle relaxant, or tranquilizer drug. One or more of these medicines may provide strong temporary relief, but none are considered safe for long-term use.

ASPIRIN: THE FIRST NON-STEROIDAL ANTI-INFLAMMATORY DRUG (NSAID)

Modern treatment of arthritis pain began with an old herbal remedy. Europeans and Native Americans had long used willow bark tea to relieve pain, with significant, albeit limited success. But this mild folk remedy turned out to be the start of something stronger, in both its pharmacological effects and its medical significance. As early as 1838, an Italian chemist managed to identify willow bark's active constituents—a family of chemicals called salicylates. The most potent analgesic compound in willow bark, called salicylic acid, proved too irritating to the stomach to be used in isolation as a synthetic drug. Then, in 1853, an Alsatian scientist synthesized acetylsalicylic acid. This chemical is just as effective as salicylic acid, but gentler on the gastrointestinal tract.

Years later, chemist Felix Hofman at Germany's Bayer drug company put his arthritic father on a regimen of acetylsalicylic acid, with great success in relieving the man's pain. By 1899, Bayer had introduced acetylsalicylic acid to the marketplace as "aspirin." Under this trade name, acetylsalicylic acid quickly went on to become the world's most widely used nonprescription arthritis drug—a double-edged sword that can accelerate tissue damage even as it relieves pain.

SYNTHETIC NSAIDs

Drug companies now produce many synthetic NSAIDs, including diclofenac, diflunisal, etodolac, flurbiprofen, ibuprofen, indomethacin, ketoprofen, nabumetone, naproxen, piroxicam, salsalate, sulindac, and trilisate. Until recently, with the development of COX-2 inhibitors like celecoxib (see "Safer New NSAIDs" in this chapter), the search for a strong, trouble-free synthetic NSAID had been largely unsuccessful. Indomethacin has a higher risk of side effects than most NSAIDs but generally produces stronger anti-inflammatory effects. It is often used as the standard against which anti-inflammatory herbs, nutritional supplements, and drugs are tested. The convenient, single-daily-dose NSAID called piroxicam (Felden) has been accused of posing greater risks of gastric damage than other NSAIDs, but available statistics do not seem to bear out this claim. Note: Never combine NSAIDs without medical guidance, and be aware that appropriate dosages vary widely among these drugs.

STINGING NETTLES FOR PAIN?
GIVING NSAIDs AN HERBAL ASSIST

Should NSAIDs fail to provide sufficient relief, there may be a way to enjoy better results without increasing your intake. Two studies indicate that extract of stinging nettle (Urtica dioica) may make low doses of NSAIDs as effective as high doses in alleviating key symptoms of rheumatoid arthritis. In the first trial, half of forty participating patients took 200 milligrams of diclofenac, a synthetic NSAID, and the other half took 50 milligrams of diclofenac plus 50 grams (1.8 ounces) of stewed nettle leaf, with equally positive results on laboratory and clinical measures (e.g., elevated levels of complement proteins and less pain, impairment, and stiffness).[1] These results support earlier findings showing that consumption of a dried, powdered extract of nettle leaf allowed participants to cut their NSAID dose by three-quarters with no loss of efficacy.[2]

SIDE EFFECTS OF ASPIRIN AND OTHER NSAIDs

Aspirin and other NSAIDs are remarkably powerful analgesics, but they produce serious adverse effects in many people. This is especially true when NSAIDs are taken at the high daily doses needed to tame serious arthritis pain, but it holds true even at fairly low doses.[3] According to 1995 testimony before the FDA, NSAIDs are estimated to cause 41,000 hospitalizations each year, the result of a variety of adverse effects.[4] Researchers have concluded that the death toll from NSAIDs is much higher than previous estimates—a staggering 16,500 additional deaths every year.[5]

FREQUENT SIDE EFFECTS

- Stomach pain, heartburn, nausea[6]
- Cartilage degeneration[7–10]
- Leaky gut syndrome (see Chapters 6 and 10)[11, 12]
- Cramping and diarrhea
- Fluid retention and weight gain
- Drowsiness, dizziness, mental fuzziness
- Wounds bleed more, heal more slowly [Note: Do not use NSAIDs or Tylenol in combination with anticoagulant

coumarin derivatives such as warfarin. Use them with caution when taking herbs containing coumarin (angelica, astragalus, celery seed, licorice, passionflower, etc.) or anticoagulant omega-3 oils from fish, flax, and hemp.]
• Adverse reactions with alcohol or vitamin C (aspirin only)
• Ringing in ears
• Lowering of nighttime melatonin levels (up to 75%) and body temperature[13]

COMMON SIDE EFFECTS

Some patients may experience gastric ulcers and/or serious gastric bleeding. In half of all people who regularly take NSAIDs, detectable erosions in the lining of the stomach or upper intestine develop, and 15–20% get ulcers.[14,15] Even at low daily doses (325 milligrams), aspirin triples the risk of bleeding. A smaller percentage of patients experience bleeding or perforated ulcers. One two-year scientific survey of 1,900 people who routinely used NSAIDs showed that 80% of those who had potentially fatal gastric bleeding noticed no warning symptoms.[16]

RARE SIDE EFFECTS

• Anemia from bleeding ulcers
• Infertility in men and women[17]
• Liver or kidney damage

A team at Johns Hopkins University questioned 716 men and women with serious kidney damage who were undergoing regular dialysis. For comparison, they also interviewed a control group of 316 people from the general population. All were asked about their past use of NSAIDs and acetaminophen. People with end-stage kidney disease were more likely to report a high level of lifetime consumption of NSAIDs and acetaminophen, with acetaminophen producing the highest risk. Surprisingly, the controls with healthy kidneys reported having taken a greater total amount of aspirin in their lives, in comparison with the kidney patients. This result suggests that NSAIDs may be safer than acetaminophen with respect to the kidneys.[18]

COUNTERING NSAID SIDE EFFECTS

The serious gastric effects of NSAIDs prevent many people from being able to tolerate effective doses over the long term. The proportion of arthritis patients who have ulcers (15–20%) far exceeds the proportion of the general population (1–3%), and about one in three older arthritis patients suffers ulcers from NSAIDs.[19-21] To limit gastric side effects, first find the NSAID(s) that cause you the least stomach upset. Try to take the drugs with meals and cut back on irritating foods and drinks, such as alcohol, coffee, and chocolate. You can also take some NSAIDs in special forms that may reduce gastric discomfort (see "Safer New NSAIDs" in this chapter). As a last resort, antacids and new antiulcer drugs may allow you to better tolerate gastric side effects.

About one in three people who take NSAIDs daily also take an antacid or acid-blocker drug. The Stanford University study cited earlier found, however, that these drugs may increase the danger from NSAIDs by masking the development of bleeding ulcers. In fact, arthritis patients who routinely consume antacids or acid-blockers suffer gastric complications twice as often as those who take them only periodically, in response to gastric symptoms.[22] There are several options for countering the side effects of NSAIDs—none of which is entirely effective or free of its own side effects:

Enteric coatings lessen but do not eliminate gastric irritation or ulcers, by delaying release of the drug until it reaches the small intestines. **Time-release NSAIDs** maintain steadier blood levels of the drug over time. Like enteric coatings, time-release pills decrease but do not eliminate the risk of gastric irritation or ulcers. **Soft aspirin tablets** cut the risk of gastric irritation or ulcers by speeding dissolution and absorption of the drug.

Buffered aspirin neutralizes stomach acids and may minimize upsets, but it will not prevent gastric irritation or ulcers. New research confirms that buffered aspirin does not lower the risk of gastrointestinal bleeding. In fact, when comparing their effects at equivalently high doses, the risk of bleeding is slightly higher for buffered than for plain aspirin.[23]

Antacids, such as Rolaids, Tums, and Mylanta, neutralize stomach acid. They can cause diarrhea or constipation and can interfere with absorption of other medications, including tetracycline.

Histamine H$_2$ antagonists limit the production of stomach acid. These antagonists include ranitidine (Zantac) and cimetidine (Tagamet). To the extent that rheumatoid arthritis can be promoted by leaky gut syndrome (see Chapters 6 and 10), it may be counterproductive for rheumatic patients to overuse these drugs. Each is associated with numerous potential side effects, including, in the case of cimetidine, joint pain. Moreover, a Stanford University research team found that H$_2$ acid-blockers "may actually increase the probability of a serious event by creating a false sense of security for the physician and the patient."[24]

Two new studies indicate that **omeprazole (Prilosec)**—one in a new class of drugs called acid pump inhibitors—is the most effective treatment for ulcers caused by NSAIDs. In one study, Prilosec improved ulcers and pre-ulcerous erosions within eight weeks in 80% of 541 participants, compared with 63% who took Zantac. Prilosec continued to perform better during a six-month follow-up. In a second study, Prilosec outperformed misoprostol. Among nine hundred participants, 61% enjoyed improvement while on Prilosec versus 48% on misoprostol, and Prilosec produced fewer of the adverse effects—mostly diarrhea and stomach pain—that people experienced with both drugs.[25]

One study of nine thousand rheumatoid arthritis patients indicates that misoprostol (Cytotec), a **synthetic prostaglandin,** can minimize intestinal side effects of NSAIDs by up to 40%.[26] Misoprostol decreases production of gastric acid and increases production of gastric mucus. Ironically, it can also cause adverse gastrointestinal and menstrual side effects, among others. Arthrotec, a new drug approved in dozens of countries, combines the NSAID diclofenac and misoprostol in one pill. As of this writing, Arthrotec was under review by the FDA, with approval expected before 1999.

Sucralfate coats ulcers to protect them from acid, helping them resist further damage. Not an antacid, sucralfate reduces absorption of cimetidine, ranitidine, and others and must be taken two hours before these medications.

COUNTERPRODUCTIVE
EFFECTS OF NSAIDs

Too often, doctors fail to mention that use of NSAIDs makes matters worse. NSAIDs hinder construction of the chemical building blocks of cartilage and may also increase their natural rate of decay.[27–32] There is no serious scientific controversy over these startling facts, yet you will find no such warnings on NSAID product labels, and you may not hear them from your doctor either.

When doctors had no other treatment to offer, it might have been reasonable to downplay this seriously counterproductive side effect of NSAIDs, if not the potential for ulcers and even death. Some may have considered it pointless to make patients anxious about the safety of the only pain relief then available. As we will see in Chapter 4, viable new options for treating the pain and progressive damage of osteoarthrosis demand a more balanced view of the risks of long-term use of NSAIDs.

It is important to point out that some NSAIDs do more cartilage damage than others. One study has examined the effects of various NSAIDs on cartilage taken from 150 patients.[33] The results showed that NSAIDs can be divided into three categories based on their ability to reduce the body's production of cartilage components called glycosaminoglycans, or GAGs (see Chapter 4). In the first category, naproxen, ibuprofen, and indomethacin cause significant damage. Much less damage is affected by aspirin, piroxicam, diclofenac, and tiaprofenic acid, while aceclofenac, tenidap, and tolmetin have entirely insignificant effects.

HOW NSAIDs HELP AND HURT

Aspirin and other NSAIDs suppress inflammation and alleviate the pain it causes. For many years, science did not know how NSAIDs work. Today we have a better picture of how NSAIDs suppress inflammation and pain. This information is stimulating efforts to develop safer synthetic NSAIDs and is critical to an understanding of the safe, effective natural alternatives that are currently available (see Chapters 11 and 12).

IMMUNE CELLS INITIATE INFLAMMATION

The human immune system consists primarily of several types of white blood cells. Each of these "immune cells" performs unique functions in response to injuries or infections. Some immune cells initiate inflammatory "cascade reactions," which yield hormonelike chemical messengers that increase the pressure, thickness, and flow of blood around injured or infected tissue. This results in the swelling, heat, redness, and pain associated with inflamed tissues.

SAFER NEW NSAIDs: NATURAL AND SYNTHETIC ALTERNATIVES

The inflammatory cascade reactions initiated by immune cells produce a group of chemicals called "inflammatory mediators"—primarily **leukotrienes** and certain **prostaglandins**. All of the various NSAIDs work by hindering the action of enzymes needed to ignite inflammatory cascade reactions. (NSAIDs may also work by blocking the B vitamin called folic acid, which would hinder immune cells' ability to initiate inflammatory cascade reactions.[34]) One pair of cascade reactions in particular yields many of the inflammatory mediators at work in arthritis. These cascade reactions—called COX-1 and COX-2—are named after the cyclooxygenase (COX) enzymes that ignite them.[35] Most NSAIDs produce their analgesic effects by blocking both of these COX enzymes and the inflammatory cascade reactions they facilitate.

One of these inflammatory mediators—COX-1—serves several other important metabolic functions. When the COX-1 enzyme is continuously blocked (disabled) by an NSAID drug, serious side effects result. This is because the COX-1 cascade reaction governs the prostaglandin (PGI_2) that ensures adequate production of intestinal mucus, which in turn protects intestinal walls from irritating substances—including NSAIDs. Aspirin and most other synthetic NSAIDs induce gastric bleeding and upset precisely because they block the COX-1 reaction. And every year, thousands of Americans suffer or even die from silent gastric bleeding related to long-term use of NSAIDs.

NATURAL AND EXPERIMENTAL COX-2 NSAIDs

Certain herbs and "nutraceutical" food substances lessen inflammation almost as effectively as synthetic NSAIDs without producing gastric side effects (see Chapters 12 and 13). These natural substances appear to block the COX-2 cascade or other inflammatory reactions without strongly blocking the COX-1 cascade reaction—an effect that would explain why they limit inflammation and pain without the side effects typical of NSAIDs.

During the early 1990s, American inflammation expert Phillip Needleman developed a highly promising synthetic counterpart to these safer, natural NSAIDs. By examining the existing NSAIDs that did the least damage to the intestines, he developed a chemical structure that would selectively block COX-2 over COX-1. In March of 1995, Dr. Needleman's team at G. D. Searle began clinical testing of the new drug, called celecoxib (Celebra). Celecoxib blocks the COX-2 cascade one thousand times more effectively than it blocks the COX-1 cascade and reportedly produces no significant side effects. The drug has been tested against rheumatoid arthritis and osteoarthrosis and appears to be a very potent pain reliever that also improves range of motion. Pending the results of further studies, celecoxib should be approved in the United States by the end of 1999. The Merck pharmaceutical company has its own COX-2 drug, called Vioxx, which will soon offer competition to celecoxib. They may have some catching up to do, since Dr. Needleman's team has also developed a second-generation COX-2 NSAID that is forty-two times more effective than celecoxib at selectively blocking COX-2 rather than COX-1.

Natural and synthetic COX-2 blockers may be the most important breakthrough in arthritis therapy. In addition to relieving pain and inflammation very effectively with no significant side effects, these drugs may prevent much of the inflammation-inflicted tissue damage that occurs in rheumatic diseases. And discovery of COX-2 NSAIDs may represent a major breakthrough in prevention of cancer and cognitive decline in Alzheimer's disease. What is the common thread in rheumatic disease, cancer, and Alzheimer's?

Much of the damage to neuron cells in the brains of Alzheimer's patients stems from a destructive inflammatory response to neuronal damage caused by various factors. By the end of the twentieth century, a new national study will have shown whether celecoxib can, as suspected, sharply curtail the rate of mental decline among Alzheimer's patients. Colon cancer—and possibly breast cancer as well—begins with a mutation that causes cells to produce excess COX-2. This reaction gives rise to precancerous polyps that become cancerous following a second mutation. By blocking COX-2 enzymes, celecoxib may kill cancerous changes in the cradle.

ACETAMINOPHEN: PAIN RELIEF WITH THE LEADING "UN-NSAID"

As we have seen, the side effects produced by standard COX-1 NSAIDs have prompted a search for synthetic analgesics with fewer side effects. The first of these was acetaminophen. Discovered not long after aspirin was introduced by Bayer, acetaminophen (Tylenol and others) is not an anti-inflammatory drug. Instead of blocking inflammatory cascade reactions, it reduces pain by acting on the nervous system. Accordingly, acetaminophen can work well for the mechanical pain typical of osteoarthrosis, but it is considered less effective against the inflammatory pain of rheumatic diseases. On the other hand, acetaminophen does not produce the gastric symptoms associated with synthetic NSAIDs.

Acetaminophen is not without side effects. Like some NSAIDs, it can cause liver or kidney damage over the long term. The risks of acetaminophen to the liver and kidneys were evaluated at the University of Pittsburgh Medical Center. Researchers examined the records of patients with serious liver damage who also regularly used more than 4 grams of acetaminophen a day (twelve regular-strength tablets).[36] Their findings were as follows:

- People eating normally and drinking little alcohol suffered liver damage at levels of 15 grams of acetaminophen per day.
- Those who ate very little food—owing to flu, jaw injury, and so on—suffered liver damage at doses of only 4 grams per day.
- Those who drank to excess but ate normal amounts of food experienced liver damage at 10 grams per day.

Based on these results, it appears that the greatest risk from acetaminophen is associated with failure to eat enough food while taking the drug.

In the Johns Hopkins University study previously cited (see "Rare Side Effects" in this chapter), kidney failure was found to be most closely associated with a lifetime intake of five thousand or more acetaminophen pills.[37] No one should take acetaminophen or NSAIDs regularly or at higher than standard nonprescription doses except under a physician's guidance. This is especially true of people with liver damage or disease and people who drink more than one bottle of beer, one glass of wine, or one ounce of liquor per day.

CHAPTER 4

THE CARTILAGE THERAPY REVOLUTION

GLUCOSAMINE, CHONDROITIN, BOVINE CARTILAGE, SULFUR, GELATIN, BOSWELLIA HERB

PEOPLE WITH OSTEOARTHROSIS ARE OFTEN told that a gradual decline in joint health is inevitable and that they must live with pain and analgesic drugs, but this may not be true. First, there is some evidence that osteoarthrosis can slowly improve with exercise, physical therapy, and avoidance of conventional NSAIDs.[1, 2] In addition, a quiet revolution in clinical research has produced several dietary supplements that appear to halt or slow the cartilage destruction behind osteoarthrotic pain. These so-called cartilage protective agents, or CPAs, are widely used by European physicians, but they have been overlooked by American doctors. It is premature to call any CPA a "cure" for osteoarthrosis, but there is ample evidence to suggest that some CPAs may halt or even reverse joint degradation while relieving pain as effectively as most NSAIDs. Before we describe CPAs in more depth, it is important to understand the nature of cartilage and how this key connective tissue is nurtured and protected.

CARTILAGE:
CREATION AND DESTRUCTION

As we have seen, the causes of primary osteoarthrosis are uncertain, but they probably include genetic traits, aging, malnutrition, free radical stress, and repetitive stress on joints. Lacking any blood vessels, cartilage must rely on the pumping action of moving joints to transport wastes and nutrients in and out of synovial fluid. Since pain discourages the use of affected joints, it is easy to see how the downward spiral of cartilage and bone degradation described in Chapter 1 can result from injuries to joint tissues.

Aging alone does not explain most cases of osteoarthrosis. In fact, the chemical composition of cartilage in osteoarthrosis sufferers actually shifts back to the pattern seen in children.[3, 4] There is considerable evidence, however, that malnutrition, genetic factors, and aging can combine to impair the body's ability to renew the key chemical components of cartilage. Perhaps the most critical loss due to aging is the ability to make sufficient amounts of protein-sugar compounds called glycosaminoglycans—especially glucosamine sulfate, a key structural constituent of cartilage tissues. This obscure chemical may be the first therapeutic agent able to halt the cartilage destruction that underlies osteoarthrosis.[5, 6] To understand how this very promising treatment works, it helps to learn a bit about the structure of articular (joint) cartilage—a tough, cushiony matrix consisting of six elements:

- Water, which constitutes about three-quarters of the matter that makes up cartilage.
- The small building-block molecules called glycosaminoglycans. (The primary GAG molecule in cartilage is glucosamine sulfate, which constitutes 50% of hyaluronic acid.)
- Hyaluronic acid, a compound made up of linked GAGs, about half of which are glucosamine sulfate.
- Huge, treelike molecules called proteoglycans (PGs), which snake through strands of collagen protein fibers to form the

matrix that gives cartilage its remarkable strength and resiliency. Each PG molecule is organized around a central "trunk" made of hyaluronic acid, from which radiate long, branchlike protein molecules. Shorter, bristly "branches" made of chondroitin sulfate radiate from each of these main branches. Viewed through an electron microscope, proteoglycans look like spiraling, cylindrical pine trees. As people age, these trees tend to fray and lose branches and resiliency.

- Chondroitin sulfate molecules, which consist of chains (polymers) of linked glucosamine sulfate molecules.
- Tough, elastic strands of collagen (and elastin) that lend cartilage shape and amazing tensile strength.

Together, these elements provide the cushioning and gliding properties of cartilage. Both chondroitin and glucosamine possess negative electric charges, an attribute that serves two important structural functions. First, the negative charge causes proteoglycan "branches" to repel each other, thereby maintaining the open spaces between them. Second, the negative charge attracts and holds water in those spaces. This water-attracting property of GAG molecules is critical to the shock-absorbing property of cartilage. Water is squeezed out of the proteoglycan–collagen matrix by physical pressure on joints but is immediately sucked back in by its electrical attraction to GAG molecules.

Arthritis researchers now believe that decay of PGs is central to the disease process in most cases of osteoarthrosis. As people age, their proteoglycans become smaller and structure less water around themselves, in part because of the smaller size of their chondroitin sulfate chains. Inflammation or infection can produce abnormal amounts of free radicals, which degrade cartilage tissue, stimulate release of cartilage-dissolving enzymes, and decrease production of chondroitin sulfate. And the antioxidant-poor diets of most Americans leave tissues unprotected against free radical damage.

Aging, damaged, malnourished cartilage needs two things: dietary antioxidants like vitamin C and OPC (oligomeric proanthocyaniden; see Chapters 11 and 13) to neutralize free radicals and an ample supply of GAGs to construct and repair chondroitin sulfate and proteoglycans. Otherwise, cartilage will begin to fragment. You can picture joint cartilage as a water bed filled with water, a network of stiff rubber cords (collagen), and firm, shock-absorbing, cylindrical sponges (PGs)—a combination that provides cushioning and resiliency. Together, free radical stress and the aging process gradually fray and shrink the sponges, limiting their ability to hold water. When the bed can no longer support concentrated pressure, you end up perched on a hard floor. If you are overweight or are constantly jumping up and down on the bed, you will begin hitting the floor even sooner. To maintain the resiliency of cartilage, the body must be able to replace and repair chondroitin sulfate molecules and PGs. But in people with primary osteoarthrosis, the rate of decay exceeds the rate of repair.[7]

CARTILAGE PROTECTORS: TREATING ROOT CAUSES

In response to injury to cartilage, the immune cells embedded in subchondral bone release free radicals that can become a contributing factor in primary osteoarthrosis. There is ample evidence that antioxidant supplements—specifically vitamins E and C—can help protect cartilage from decaying under assault by free radicals. Nutritional therapy should probably include these nutrients and others shown to help (vitamin B_5 and B_6, zinc, and copper—see Chapter 11 for more information on nutritional intervention).

GLUCOSAMINE SULFATE: THE PRIMARY PROTECTOR

Over the past decade, researchers have made the exciting discovery that dietary supplementation with cartilage or its key chemical components can help protect or even restore damaged cartilage in animals and humans with osteoarthrosis. The key cartilage protective agents are glucosamine sulfate, chondroitin sulfate, and purified bovine (calf) cartilage. All three have been the subject of animal research and human clinical trials concerning arthritis, with encouraging results. Each of these "nutraceutical" dietary supplements is a weak anti-inflammatory agent. And, more important, they enhance the body's own efforts to repair cartilage tissues. They are available without a prescription in most health food and drug stores. Of the three, glucosamine sulfate enjoys the best scientific evidence of efficacy, followed by chondroitin sulfate and bovine cartilage.[8, 9]

There are several synthetic CPAs that may confer similar benefits, including diacerein, amprilose hydrochloride, N-acetyl glucosamine (PolyNAG) and S-adenosyl-L-methionine (SAMe). Some European countries have already approved SAMe for use in osteoarthrosis. As of this writing, none of the synthetic CPAs—except NS2 glucosamine—were available to doctors or patients in the United States. And none appears to hold as much promise as glucosamine sulfate.

Glucosamine sulfate may be the first effective, root-level remedy for osteoarthrosis. In the mid-1960s, several research teams began seeking a single constituent of animal cartilage that might be responsible for most of the potent healing properties. This work led to research on glucosamine compounds, which failed to match the healing effects of whole cartilage but still produced positive results.[10]

These findings were largely ignored by American doctors but piqued the interest of many international researchers, who went on to conduct controlled clinical trials of glucosamine sulfate in osteoarthrosis. Their remarkably uniform findings strongly suggest that glucosamine sulfate relieves pain as effectively as NSAIDs—with no significant side effects. And unlike NSAIDs, which interfere with the body's ability to repair cartilage, glucosamine sulfate enhances the natural healing process.

Despite clear, credible evidence suggesting that it may be safer and more effective than NSAIDs, North American doctors have failed to act on the strong evidence in favor of glucosamine sulfate. This failure stems from a general lack of knowledge about or interest in research conducted overseas. One American biomedical researcher expressed his dismay in blunt terms: "Medical researchers and physicians in the US have totally ignored this rational and safe therapeutic strategy."[11] Another researcher has written, "In particular glucosamine sulfate, which naturally occurs in the human body and is almost devoid of toxicity, [has] remarkable chondroprotective [cartilage-protecting] effects [and] is suitable for long-term therapeutic use."[12]

The Research: Glucosamine Sulfate on Trial

As we have seen, GAGs are needed to construct the huge PG molecules that keep cartilage firm but flexible. At the risk of oversimplifying matters, it can be said that osteoarthrosis results when the body fails to replace PGs as fast as they decay. In the 1980s, doctors looking for ways to fix this imbalance began experimenting with natural and synthetic GAGs. Researchers began putting glucosamine sulfate to the test in controlled clinical trials. In a controlled study, one group of volunteers gets the test drug, and another group of comparable size and health status receives a placebo or alternate drug of known potency. (A placebo is an inactive substance administered in a form that neither the patient nor the doctor can distinguish from the test drug.)

Most of these controlled studies also employed double-blind methodology, which means that neither the doctors nor the participants knew who was getting the test drug and who was getting a placebo or conventional NSAID. Double-blinding avoids the well-known "placebo effect," in which test subjects' symptoms recede for a time because they believe they are getting a real medicine. The international investigators soon discovered that dietary supplements containing glucosamine sulfate relieve osteoarthrosis symptoms as well as NSAIDs—at least in the short term. Better yet, they found that glucosamine sulfate works by accelerating the body's production of PGs, among other healing processes.

To date, there have been ten controlled trials of glucosamine sulfate published in respected scientific journals—seven of whose results we summarize here.[13–22] In each of the trials, glucosamine sulfate was tested against either a synthetic NSAID or a placebo. Except for the unfortunately short duration of the glucosamine trials, this is the type of clinical research that the FDA has often accepted when approving a novel synthetic drug. We have excerpted or paraphrased the dramatically positive results of several of these trials, so that you can hear from the investigators themselves.

Oral Glucosamine Sulfate Versus NSAID (Ibuprofen)

"Although the rate of decrease was slower [for the glucosamine group versus the NSAID group], the reduction in pain scores was continued throughout the trial period in patients on glucosamine and the difference between the two groups turned significantly in favour of glucosamine at Week 8 . . . with only minor complaints being reported by 2 patients on glucosamine compared with 5 patients on ibuprofen."[23]

Oral Glucosamine Sulfate Versus NSAID (Ibuprofen)

English researchers conducted a four-week-long double-blind clinical trial that pitted glucosamine sulfate against ibuprofen in 252 outpatients with active osteoarthrosis of the knee. Again, improvement was quicker during the first week for the ibuprofen group (400 milligrams twice a day). By the second week, however, the glucosamine group (500 milligrams twice a day) had caught up in terms of pain relief. While one in three of the ibuprofen group reported side effects—usually stomach upset—none of the glucosamine patients experienced any problems. The researchers concluded that glucosamine may be a safe and effective slow-acting drug for osteoarthrosis.[24]

Injected Glucosamine Sulfate Versus Placebo

"When orally given . . . [glucosamine sulfate] is more effective than placebo and at least as effective as non-steroidal anti-inflammatory drugs [NSAIDs] in osteoarthritis symptoms. The aim of this multi-centre, randomised, placebo-controlled, double-blind, parallel-group study was to assess the efficacy and safety of glucosamine sulfate intramuscularly given on the same parameters [symptoms]. A significant decrease in the [Lesquesne] index [of symptomatic severity] was observed for glucosamine compared to placebo. . . . These proportions were 51% [glucosamine sulfate] vs. 30% [placebo]."[25]

Oral Glucosamine Sulfate Versus NSAIDs and Placebo

"[For both the glucosamine and NSAID groups] each symptom improved, but to a faster and greater extent in the group treated with glucosamine. . . . A further improvement [in the second half of the test, versus placebo] was recorded in the patients treated with glucosamine. . . . It is suggested that . . . oral treatment with pure glucosamine sulphate should be considered as basic therapy for the management of primary or secondary osteoarthritis."[26]

Injected Glucosamine Sulfate Versus Placebo

"Glucosamine administration [by injection in the knee] was able to accelerate the recovery of arthrosic patients, with no resulting side effects, and to partially restore articular function. In addition, the clinical recovery did not fade after treatment ended, but lasted for the following month, at least. These features are a definite improvement over antirheumatic drugs, the major drawbacks of which are action of short duration and side effects. Glucosamine therapy therefore deserves a selected place in the management of osteoarthritis."[27]

Oral Glucosamine Sulfate Versus Placebo

"Significant alleviation of symptoms was associated with the use of the active drug [glucosamine sulfate]. . . . Use of glucosamine sulfate [as opposed to placebo] also resulted in a significantly larger proportion of patients who experienced lessening or disappearance of symptoms. . . . No adverse reactions were reported by the patients treated with glucosamine sulfate."[28]

Oral Glucosamine Sulfate Versus Piroxicam and Placebo

In a multicenter, randomized trial, 329 patients were divided into four homogeneous groups that received one of three distinct daily treatments or placebo over a period of three months: 1,500 milligrams of glucosamine sulfate, 20 milligrams of the synthetic NSAID piroxicam (Feldene), glucosamine sulfate plus piroxicam, or a placebo pill. The first group, which received only glucosamine sulfate, had the fewest side effects—even fewer than the placebo group! The authors called glucosamine sulfate a safe, effective drug for osteoarthritis and noted "a steadily increasing effect that persisted after drug withdrawal."[29]

Glucosamine: The Orphan Arthritis Drug

The question naturally arises, "If glucosamine sulfate is so promising, why haven't I heard about it?" Word is getting out, and some progressive physicians already prescribe it for osteoarthrosis. But glucosamine's apparent value far exceeds its fame. This surprising state of affairs is the sad consequence of defects in U.S. laws governing drugs and dietary supplements.

What are these regulatory defects? Start with the fact that any natural substance that is first sold as a dietary supplement cannot then be excluded from the marketplace simply because someone later gains FDA approval to sell it as a drug. Since glucosamine sulfate is already being sold as a dietary supplement, any company selling it as an approved arthritis drug would face an identical but far less expensive competitor. As a result, drug companies have little or no financial incentive to spend the tens to hundreds of millions of dollars it would take to turn glucosamine sulfate into an FDA-approved drug.

One might expect that doctors would be so eager to offer patients safe, effective products that glucosamine sulfate would be their treatment of choice. But only approved osteoarthrosis drugs benefit from the extensive advertising directed at doctors and patients and generate routine prescriptions. Absent the extensive marketing campaigns that accompany the release of new drugs—and the professional "cover" provided by FDA approval—most physicians have studiously ignored glucosamine sulfate.

In addition, health management organizations and other managed health care plans sharply restrict the list of drugs approved for prescription, making almost no provision for promising dietary supplements. With more and more doctors working for managed care plans, patients' chances of receiving glucosamine sulfate from their doctors are not likely to increase.

Glucosamine Sulfate Versus Other GAGs

In addition to glucosamine sulfate, the dietary supplement marketplace also offers glucosamine hydrochloride and *N*-acetyl glucosamine (PolyNAG). These chemicals, however, have not been tested in arthritis patients, and it is doubtful that they offer the therapeutic value of glucosamine sulfate. Neither contains sulfur, which is a critical structural component in GAG molecules. Research performed in the 1930s indicated that arthritis patients have lower than average blood levels of sulfur and that sulfur supplementation may relieve symptoms.[30–32] (As we will see, special sulfur compounds are being sold as cartilage protective treatments for osteoarthrosis.) Finally, PolyNAG is absorbed only half as well as glucosamine sulfate and does not stimulate synthesis of GAGs.[33–36]

CHONDROITIN SULFATE: GLUCOSAMINE'S PERFECT PARTNER?

Some doctors recommend taking dietary supplements of chondroitin sulfate in addition to glucosamine sulfate. The former is a water-attracting/binding compound made up of dozens of GAGs, including glucosamine sulfate. Controlled clinical studies of oral and injected doses of chondroitin sulfate—five, to date—have produced results that are quite good, but weaker than those seen with glucosamine sulfate.[37–41] The four studies that involved oral administration of chondroitin sulfate employed daily doses totaling 800–1,200 milligrams.

In one placebo-controlled trial of 120 osteoarthrosis patients, most were able to significantly limit but not eliminate their use of NSAIDs. Those receiving chondroitin sulfate also showed objective signs of substantial symptomatic relief, with none reporting serious adverse effects.[42]

GLUCOSAMINE SULFATE VERSUS CHONDROITIN SULFATE

Glucosamine and chondroitin sulfate perform complementary functions in cartilage, and some researchers believe that it makes sense to take both. This view is supported by experiments in test tubes and animals that produced results superior to using glucosamine alone. Glucosamine sulfate effects very good clinical results by itself, however, and is considerably less costly. There are a number of reasons to believe that chondroitin has little to add to glucosamine's value as a therapeutic agent.

Certainly, chondroitin sulfate performs critical metabolic functions with obvious therapeutic applications. Like glucosamine sulfate, it attracts vital water into the cartilage matrix and stimulates production of key cartilage constituents (GAGs, PGs, collagen). And, unlike glucosamine sulfate, chondroitin sulfate has the ability to prevent enzymes from dissolving cartilage and robbing it of nutrients.[43–45]

Chondroitin sulfate, however, produces markedly weaker clinical results than glucosamine sulfate. This may be due in part to its much larger molecular size, which greatly lessens the amount absorbed (0–13% versus 90–98% of glucosamine sulfate).[46–48] Your body does not need supplemental chondroitin to make more, since it is made up of linked glucosamine sulfate molecules. Moreover, glucosamine sulfate alone stimulates synthesis of chondroitin by cartilage cells (chondrocytes). Finally, chondroitin sulfate has been subjected to far fewer clinical trials, and in most of them, positive results were achieved with injections of the molecule—a costly, uncomfortable, time-consuming method. These factors explain why most practitioners recommend taking glucosamine alone for eight weeks, to see whether benefit is achieved before adding the expense of supplemental chondroitin sulfate.

BOVINE CARTILAGE:
THE ORIGINAL CPA

Animal cartilage has been used to accelerate healing of damaged human cartilage since World War I, but scientific confirmation of the unique healing powers of animal cartilage had to wait forty years. In 1957, Drs. John F. Prudden and Gentaro Mishihara published a scientific article entitled "The Acceleration of Wound Healing with Cartilage-1." A follow-up controlled clinical study, published in the May 1965 issue of the *Journal of the American Medical Association,* confirmed their findings. Since then, bovine cartilage has become an accepted part of the modern medical repertoire, used to speed healing of connective tissues damaged by injury or surgery.

Dr. Prudden became interested in the obvious possibility that cartilage might be useful in treating diseases of connective tissues—especially osteoarthrosis and rheumatic forms of arthritis. He set out to see if the anti-inflammatory, wound-healing properties he and others had already documented for a purified bovine cartilage product (Catrix) could help in combating osteoarthrosis. (No animals are killed to make bovine cartilage products, since it comes from animals raised for their meat.) As Dr. Prudden wrote in 1974, "The assumptions were that a reconstitution of the affected cartilage might well be achieved by furnishing biochemical components that could be utilized in resynthesis [of chondroitin sulfates] and that the anti-inflammatory effect would be of benefit."[49] Three subsequent experiments—one using injected cartilage and two employing oral cartilage—found that this approach could be remarkably effective.

Injected Cartilage: Uncontrolled Study

In an uncontrolled study conducted by Dr. Prudden and associates at Columbia University, Catrix was tested as an injectable treatment for osteoarthrosis. Of twenty-eight subjects with severe osteoarthrosis, 67% enjoyed excellent results, and 21% experienced good results. Each received injections of Catrix solution (300–800 milliliters) over periods ranging from three to eight weeks. Remarkably, relief lasted for an average of seven months after treatment stopped. There were no side effects reported, and no signs of toxicity showed up in extensive lab tests.[50]

Oral Cartilage: Uncontrolled Study

Dr. Prudden then tested the effects of oral cartilage in seven hundred osteoarthrosis patients. Each patient was given nine grams of Catrix per day; of the 700 patients, 85% reported good or excellent results. The duration of benefit was quite a bit shorter than for injectable Catrix—about three weeks of improvement after cessation of oral therapy versus several months of improvement after cessation of injection therapy.[51] Incredibly, none of this work was followed up by arthritis researchers.

Oral Cartilage: Placebo-Controlled Five-Year Study

The only other clinical trial of oral bovine cartilage in osteoarthrosis—conducted at Charles University Medical School in Prague, Czechoslovakia—lasted much longer and produced equally impressive results. Pain scores for 147 osteoarthrosis patients who received bovine cartilage dropped an average of 85% after sixty days (versus only 5% in the placebo group). And, significantly, subjects receiving bovine cartilage had 37% less joint degeneration over the five-year period of the trial.[52]

Dr. Prudden believes that patients may benefit from taking both glucosamine sulfate and cartilage. As he said during a recent telephone interview, "It seems likely that glucosamine is a key constituent in bovine cartilage as far as cartilage repair goes. But glucosamine is very soluble and is excreted rapidly through the kidneys. Ideally, we need something that gives a slower release. It may make sense to take bovine cartilage and glucosamine together, to take advantage of the strengths of each—more consistent efficacy from glucosamine sulfate and slow release of GAGs from bovine cartilage."[53]

Shark Cartilage: CPA from the Sea?

Shark cartilage may be an effective alternative to bovine cartilage for treating osteoarthrosis, because its chemical constituents and biological effects are similar to those of bovine cartilages. But claims made for shark cartilage rest almost entirely on clinical trials using bovine cartilage. There are several factors to consider when deciding between bovine and shark cartilage.

- Shark cartilage has not been tested in any published, peer-reviewed clinical trials relating to arthritis. In a small eight-week study, Dr. Jose Orcasita of the University of Miami reported significant pain relief in five of six participants, but at very high daily doses of shark cartilage—8,880 milligrams, or about one-third of an ounce per day.
- Measured by weight, bovine cartilage contains about twice as much of each of the constituents proved to promote healthy cartilage—GAGs and chondroitin sulfate. In addition, bovine cartilage costs considerably less than shark cartilage gram for gram.
- The bovine cartilage products introduced to the marketplace to date have been purified, sterile supplements manufactured to pharmaceutical specifications. Brands of shark cartilage range more widely in reliability, with those used in FDA drug trials presumably offering assured quality and safety. (Contact the maker to inquire.)
- As the Audubon Society, the World Wildlife Fund (WWF), and others have pointed out, many species of shark are becoming endangered. In 1997, a WWF report titled "An Overview of World Trade in Sharks" stated that thirty to seventy million sharks are killed annually to supply the trade in shark products, including cartilage. Sharks are on the top of the marine food

chain, and there is widespread concern among marine biologists that current over-harvesting will upset the oceans' delicate ecological balance.

- Bovine cartilage is a by-product of the beef industry. Accordingly, its production adds no independent environmental impacts.

MSM AND DMSO: THE SULFUR CONNECTION

Sulfur is an essential component in the GAG compounds that constitute most cartilage tissue, and arthritis patients are often lacking in this overlooked element. Despite sulfur's key role in cartilage, its therapeutic potential has gone relatively unexamined. The success of glucosamine sulfate may gain it more attention, since many believe that its beneficial effects are traceable to its sulfur content. Two other sulfur compounds—methylsulfonylmethane (MSM) and dimethyl sulfoxide (DMSO)—have drawn attention as potential arthritis remedies. While neither appears to hold as much promise, each is worth serious examination and consideration in individual cases.

MSM: A Natural Sulfur "Donor"

MSM is a natural constituent of the human body, and traces are present in many fruits, grains, and vegetables. Supplemental MSM is a donor of sulfur atoms, which the body uses to construct cartilage constituents (GAGs), enzymes, and many other beneficial compounds. This explains why MSM has been successfully used to protect against wind and sunburn, make skin more supple, and accelerate wound healing. Our research uncovered no test tube, animal, or clinical studies showing any benefit in osteoarthrosis.

MSM seems to have gained popularity as an arthritis treatment based solely on manufacturers' vigorous promotional efforts and published anecdotal reports that it relieves arthritis pain. MSM may indeed provide benefit in osteoarthrosis, but as yet there is no evidence for this claim.

DMSO: Solvent or Sulfurous Savior?

DMSO is a sulfur compound with potent free radical scavenging properties. Used primarily as an industrial solvent, DMSO is FDA-approved for treatment of a rare form of cystitis. But DMSO has also developed a folk reputation as something of a cure-all, able to ease the pain of a variety of conditions. In the body, DMSO breaks down into MSM and other sulfur compounds. Indeed, one of the drug's characteristic effects is that is makes people's breath, and even their skin, smell strongly of garlic. (Garlic's odor comes from its many sulfur compounds.)

Anecdotal reports of DMSO's alleged analgesic powers abound. It is a fact that DMSO has antioxidant, antibacterial, and anti-inflammatory properties. A few experiments enlisting a handful of rheumatoid arthritis patients showed that injections of DMSO can lessen inflammation in synovial fluid and that DMSO can heal fibroid scar tissue buildup in kidneys—a very serious condition called secondary amyloidosis. In animal tests, however, administration of DMSO by injection and topical application does not consistently suppress inflammation or symptoms of rheumatoid arthritis. And, in one experiment using rabbits, DMSO actually worsened inflammatory damage to arthritic joint tissues. While DMSO is generally considered safe to take in the recommended doses, it has produced serious side effects in two reported cases. In one, injections of DMSO may have made an elderly person very ill. In another, topical application of DMSO by an elderly man appeared to produce serious nerve damage.

A JELL-O OPTION
FOR ARTHRITIC JOINTS?

The latest entrant into the cartilage protective field—the gelatin in products like Jell-O—can appear a bit humorous at first blush. The makers of gelatin supplements like NutraJoint and Arthred make serious claims about the capacity of their products to stimulate production of collagen in joint cartilage. Gelatin is the layperson's term for purified animal collagen—a safe, convenient source of amino acids the body uses to make collagen (i.e., hydroxyproline, glycine, arginine, proline, hydroxylysine).

Does this approach make sense? It has been proved that dietary gelatin has a positive effect on hair and nail growth, and a handful of clinical studies from Europe indicate that it can minimize pain of osteoarthrosis and related conditions.[54-58] Most of these clinical trials employed gelatin products that also contain such complementary collagen-synthesis promoters as vitamin A, glycine, and L-cystine. Nabisco, the maker of Knox gelatin, mounted a clinical trial of NutraJoint (gelatin plus vitamin C) that studied 372 patients, but the results are not yet available.

The results of one well-controlled trial are representative. Dr. Milan Adam of Prague's Institute of Rheumatism Research tested the effects of three different gelatin preparations against a placebo (egg protein) in fifty-two patients with osteoarthrosis of the hip or knee.[59] As Dr. Adam reported in 1991, "Under therapy with the substances containing gelatin, the status of pain was found to have improved in nearly all cases by the end of the respective study period . . . and in a substantially reduced need for analgesics." No changes were seen in joint structure, blood measures of inflammation, or flexibility. The greatest reductions in participants' need for NSAIDs were seen with a purified, hydrolyzed collagen product (Gelita-Sol).

It is difficult to say how gelatin stacks up against glucosamine sulfate, since they have never been tested against each other. Each product provides nutritional support to a key part of cartilage structure—proteoglycans in the case of glucosamine and collagen in the case of gelatin. Until there has been more research, it makes sense to try the better-documented glucosamine option first and add or substitute a gelatin (hydrolyzed collagen) product if the results are disappointing.

A POTENTIAL HERBAL PROTECTOR

Chemicals called boswellic acids, found in Indian frankincense *(Boswellia serrata)*, may help prevent the cartilage degradation associated with osteoarthrosis. In animal studies, boswellic acids have been shown to limit excessive loss of GAGs from cartilage—an effect that may or may not occur in humans.[60] In addition, the results of limited clinical research indicate that boswellic acids can rival the anti-inflammatory action of NSAIDs, without their side effects. Turn to Chapter 12 for more information on this promising herbal alternative to synthetic NSAIDs.

CHAPTER 5

GOUT

ONCE THOUGHT TO BE A RESULT OF GLUTTONY, gout is a metabolic disease that arises from an excess of monosodium urate (MSU) in the blood. This condition, called hyperuricemia, can produce secondary osteoarthrosis over time. Hyperuricemia affects many more people than experience symptoms of gout—a painful condition that afflicts some two million Americans, 80–90% being men over 30 and closer to 60 years of age. Hyperuricemia causes sharp MSU crystals to collect in synovial (joint) fluid and/or tendons and bursa. Half of all cases begin in the first big toe joint, followed in frequency by gout in the ankles, instep, knees, wrists, or elbows. Often, gout makes its presence felt with an acute attack of pain in one or two joints or the appearance of lumps of MSU crystals called "tophi" under the skin around the elbows, heels, and ears. Tophi may appear as lesions on radiography before they become noticeable. Joint infections and rheumatoid arthritis closely mimic the symptoms of gout—lab tests can help reveal the true cause.

"Pseudogout" is a similar but less common disorder that results from deposition of calcium crystals in joints. It progresses in a fashion similar to gout and can mimic symptoms of rheumatoid arthritis. Pseudogout occurs equally in men and women and affects about half of all people who reach age 90.

WHAT CAUSES GOUT?

Gout can be caused by long-term diuretic therapy for hypertension, use of certain medicines (including aspirin), or diets rich in a protein called purine, which yields MSU when metabolized. Gout usually arises naturally, however, as the result of one or more of three inherited tendencies:

- The body produces too little of the enzymes needed to metabolize MSU acid efficiently.
- Impaired kidney function prevents excretion of excess serum MSU.
- The body produces too much purine.

Attacks are often precipitated by high consumption of alcohol. Ironically, salicylate drugs, such as aspirin and certain other NSAIDs, hinder recovery by impairing excretion of MSU from the blood. Other risk factors include obesity, elevated blood fats, cancer, toxic chemotherapy drugs, psoriasis, and sickle cell or other hemolytic anemias.

PROGRESSION

Left untreated, the initial attack of gout usually subsides in several days, and a few people never experience another attack. But in more than 90% of cases, gout will return every few months in the form of longer-lasting attacks that may spread to other joints. As a result, early treatment is required to avoid crippling damage to joints.

DIAGNOSIS

Because the signs and progression of gout are quite distinctive, an experienced practitioner can often make a reasonably reliable diagnosis based on a patient's symptoms and history. But he or she will probably order lab tests to look for confirming signs, including excess uric acid in the blood and MSU crystals in synovial fluid.

DRUG THERAPY FOR ACUTE AND CHRONIC GOUT

Aspirin aggravates gout by raising uric acid levels. Instead, acetaminophen and nonsalicylate NSAIDs (ibuprofen, etc.) may be safely prescribed to aid in the relief of acute gout pain. To relieve the pain of gout even more effectively, doctors usually prescribe colchicine—a synthetic drug dating back to 1763. Colchicine is the active constituent in meadow saffron *(Colchicum autumnale)*, the first medicine for gout. Colchicine dampens inflammation by suppressing immune cell attacks on the uric crystals. Colchicine is highly effective but significantly toxic. The drug often provides dramatic relief in one or two days, but it may produce significant side effects, including nausea, vomiting, abdominal pain, anemia, diarrhea, hives, rashes, and hair loss. In fact, healers of an earlier era took nausea as a sign that meadow saffron was beginning to work. Given the chemical's toxicity, it is much safer to use precise doses of synthetic colchicine, rather than meadow saffron extracts of uncertain potency.

Once acute symptoms have abated, doctors typically recommend drugs that lower blood levels of MSU and thereby keep gout from persisting. Allopurinol works by blocking xanthine oxidase, the enzyme needed to produce uric acid, thereby limiting the formation of blood MSU into crystals. Sulfinpyrazone and probenecid work by enhancing excretion of MSU through the kidneys. Some of these anti-MSU drugs exacerbate gout and must be suspended during the course of an attack. Doctors may continue prescribing colchicine to control symptoms while giving the anti-MSU drugs time to work. All of the standard anti-MSU drugs come replete with contraindications and the potential for serious side effects, providing ample incentive to consider safer alternatives or adjuncts that allow you to avoid standard gout drugs or at least take less of them. There are no equivalent drugs for pseudogout, whose pain is usually treated by administration of colchicine or various NSAIDs.

DIET AND NATURAL REMEDIES

Despite their side effects, synthetic drugs became the standard medical response to gout because they can provide fast relief from excruciating pain. There are, however, promising natural remedies that may work and will not produce side effects. There may be no effective natural treatments for pseudogout, other than natural NSAIDs (see Chapters 11 and 12). Alcohol consumption often brings on attacks of gout pain, and in many cases abstention is enough to halt further attacks. But once the immediate attack has been controlled, few doctors encourage significant dietary changes. They assume that potentially curative low-purine/low-protein diets will not work or will not be followed by patients.

In defense of doctors' skeptical attitude toward dietary therapies, even strict limits on protein intake have little effect on blood levels of uric acid. Since Hippocrates' time, however, doctors have occasionally been able to cure gout by prescribing alcohol-free diets high in water (to dilute uric acid), whole grains, vegetables, and fruit and low in animal foods. It makes sense to adopt such a diet while using other therapies. While only 10–20% of the purine circulating in blood comes from foods, it is a good idea to eliminate purine-rich foods—primarily shellfish, yeast, mackerel, anchovies, sardines, organs (e.g., liver), and meats—and to limit overall protein intake. This could make the difference between gout and symptom-free hyperuricemia. Just be aware that most people need to eat about 1.3 ounces of protein per 100 pounds of body weight each day to meet their daily nutritional requirements.

NATURAL DRUGS

Like the drug allopurinol, the bioflavonoid (antioxidant plant pigment) called "quercetin" has been shown to block xanthine oxidase, the enzyme needed to produce uric acid.[1] Folic acid may be an even stronger inhibitor of xanthine oxidase and another good alternative to allopurinol. In one uncontrolled study, using dosages of 10 to 40 milligrams per day, the B vitamin provided encouraging benefits; however, further research is needed to confirm those results.[2, 3] Cautions: The very high doses of folic acid (more than 10 milligrams per day) used successfully against gout appear to be safe, but they can mask dangerous vitamin B_{12} deficiencies.[4, 5] This is a special concern for people eating antigout diets low in animal foods. People should take high doses of folic acid only under a doctor's supervision and should take supplemental B_{12} at the official U.S. Recommended Daily Value level (6 micrograms per day). In rare instances, people have exhibited allergic reactions to supplemental folic acid, with symptoms including hives, light-headedness, and difficulty in breathing (perhaps because foods with folic acid contain a chain of amino acids that slows metabolism of the vitamin).

MEDICINAL FOODS

In one study, uric acid levels dropped significantly in sufferers who consumed the equivalent of 8 ounces of cherries per day. It may be that flavonoids in the fruit produce an effect similar to that of quercetin.[6]

HERBS FOR GOUT

Aside from meadow saffron, the source of colchicine, there appear to be no proven herbal remedies for gout. Meadow root *(Filipendula ulmaria)* contains the aspirinlike compound salicylaldehyde, which is reputed to help in clearing uric acid from the blood. But skepticism is in order, since the related salicylate compound in aspirin raises blood levels of uric acid. Do not confuse meadow root with meadowsweet *(Spiraea ularia)*, whose high levels of vitamin C may actually raise uric acid levels, or with colchicine-rich meadow saffron *(Colchicum autumnale)*, which should be used only with competent herbal guidance and medical supervision. One study showed that devil's claw root extract lowers levels of uric acid in the blood and may thus be useful in cases of gout (see Chapter 12).[7]

RATIONAL DOSES: FOLIC ACID, QUERCETIN, CHERRIES, DEVIL'S CLAW

These natural alternatives, which are listed in descending order of presumed effectiveness, may relieve symptoms. Do not forget to drink 64 ounces of water every day, to dilute and flush out uric acid.

- Folic acid: Take up to 5 milligrams per day—not the usual microgram dose recommended for essential nutritional needs—with 6 micrograms of vitamin B_{12}. High doses of folic acid—that is, anything over 800 micrograms (0.8 milligrams)—should be taken only under the close supervision of a medical doctor. As noted, one successful clinical trial employed a higher dose of 10 to 40 milligrams per day, but some experts recommend starting with a lower dose.
- Quercetin: Take 1,200 milligrams per day between meals (400 milligrams three times a day).
- Cherries: Take 8 ounces per day.
- Devil's claw: Take 1,500 milligrams per day (500 milligrams three times a day).

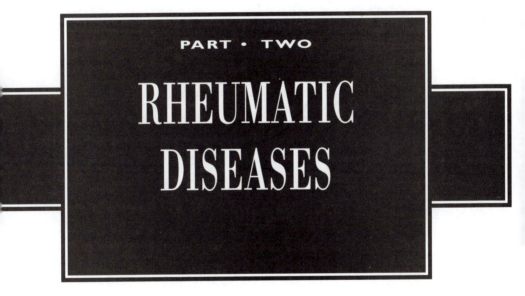

PART · TWO

RHEUMATIC DISEASES

CHAPTER 6

RHEUMATIC DISEASES

WHAT, HOW, AND WHY

IN THIS CHAPTER, WE WILL REVIEW THE DIAGNOSIS, progression, prognosis, and causes of rheumatic diseases, focusing on rheumatoid arthritis. A dozen or more connective tissue conditions, most with autoimmune aspects and inflammatory symptoms, are lumped together as "rheumatic diseases." Our chart provides an overview of the major rheumatic diseases. Compared with heart disease or cancer, these serious disorders have never attracted attention commensurate with their impact on up to ten million Americans.

Why don't rheumatic diseases make more of an impact on public awareness? Compared with cancer or heart disease, fewer people are afflicted by any one of the rheumatic diseases or are close to someone who is. Moreover, the public is generally unaware that rheumatic disorders are so debilitating, painful, and life threatening. Instead, most view "rheumatism" as a relatively trivial problem of old age—an erroneous perception that shortchanges the seriousness of these closely related conditions.

DIAGNOSIS OF RHEUMATIC DISEASES

Left untreated, most rheumatic diseases can result in serious damage to joints or internal organs. It is critical to get a proper diagnosis, which, despite today's sophisticated technologies, is easier said than done. In fact, it can be quite difficult to diagnose rheumatic diseases correctly in the first weeks or months after symptoms appear. Rheumatoid arthritis is the most common form, and doctors usually seek to eliminate or confirm it before exploring other rheumatic diagnoses. Accordingly, we will concentrate on the diagnostic procedures for this condition. In the absence of obvious, unique symptoms of other rheumatic diseases, elimination or confirmation of rheumatoid arthritis is a common starting place in the search for the correct diagnosis.

Even the most experienced rheumatologist can mistake rheumatoid arthritis for related conditions, including osteoarthrosis, ankylosing spondylitis, lupus, Reiter's disease, gout, or pseudogout. The patient's perception of pain may not be confirmed by physical examination of the joints or by blood tests and radiography, although these tests can eliminate some of the other rheumatic diseases. Normally, the examining physician will interview you to determine your symptoms and conduct a thorough, hands-on physical exam. If all or most of the following symptoms are present, it is fairly likely that the problem is rheumatoid arthritis:

- Painful joints that are red, warm, and/or tender to the touch (joints most commonly affected include finger, wrist, knee, ankle, and/or toe joints, usually on both sides of the body)

- Stiffness following periods of immobility (sleeping, sitting, etc.), which gradually improves with movement

- Inexplicable periods of fatigue or weakness

- Minor fevers, anemia, loss of appetite, weight loss

- Rheumatoid nodules (lumps of inflamed cells) under the skin

THE RHEUMATIC DISEASES[1]

Rheumatic Disease	People Affected	Typical Symptoms
Rheumatoid Arthritis	• Up to three million Americans, three-quarters of them female • Most patients develop symptoms between the ages of 25 and 50	• Inflamed joints, usually wrists, hands, shoulders, knees, and/or ankles • Affects joints symmetrically (both sides of the body) • Fatigue, morning stiffness, irritability, flulike symptoms • Rheumatoid nodules (bumps under the skin)
Ankylosing Spondylitis	• 400,000 adult Americans, three-quarters of them male • Symptoms often appear by age 30	• Dull or tender pain in the lower back, rib joints, neck, back, or shoulders, with low-grade inflammation • Potential for spinal or hip bones to fuse together • General fatigue, fever, stiffness • Pain where tendons attach to bone (ankles, buttocks, knees, and shoulders) • Iritis (eye inflammation)
Juvenile Rheumatoid Arthritis (three types, from mild to severe, with overlapping symptoms)	• 300,000 American children, three-quarters of them female	• Rheumatoid arthritis joint symptoms ranging from mild to severe • Inflammations in kidneys, heart, liver, spleen, lymph nodes • Fever, "wandering" rashes, fatigue • May have mobile nodules under skin
Psoriatic Arthritis (three types)	• 150,000 Americans— limited to 5–8% of people with psoriasis, mostly women between 20 and 30 years of age	• Red, scaly patches or sterile pustules on skin (psoriasis) • Enlarged fingers and/or toes or, more rarely, spondylitis

Rheumatic Disease	People Affected	Typical Symptoms
Psoriatic Arthritis (continued)		• Fatigue and other systemic symptoms, as in rheumatoid arthritis
Systemic Lupus Erythematosus (SLE or Lupus)	• 240,000 Americans, 90% female under age 30 • Women of African, Hispanic, and Asian background are affected five times more frequently	• Moderate joint inflammations plus autoimmune attacks on the kidneys, lungs, liver, spleen, blood vessels • Butterfly-shaped rash on face
Polymyalgia Rheumatica (PMR)	• 450,000 Americans, mostly female over age 50 • Women of Caucasian background are affected more frequently	• Pain and stiffness in the neck, shoulders, upper arms, lower back, hips, and thighs affecting both sides of the body equally • 10–50% also have giant-cell ateritis (inflamed arteries)

Let us take a quick look at the diagnostic tests that are routinely performed, plus a new one—for hemachromatosis—that is not, but probably should be. **Rheumatoid factor** is an antibody (altered gamma globulin) found in about 85% of people with rheumatoid arthritis. Tests measuring blood levels of rheumatoid factor give confirmation of a diagnosis based on physical symptoms. The **erythrocyte sedimentation rate** (ESR) provides a gauge of inflammation by measuring the speed at which red blood cells settle in solution. A high ESR means faster settling, indicating greater inflammation caused by certain blood proteins. The ESR test is useful mainly for gauging the effectiveness of anti-inflammatory therapies. Some 90% of rheumatoid arthritis patients have an elevated ESR.

Synovial fluid examination can reveal the presence of abnormally thick, cloudy synovial fluid and large numbers of neutrophils and lymphocytes (T cells)—the immune cells that typically congregate in affected joints. This exam, which requires insertion of a needle into the joint space, is also used to eliminate the possibility of gout or infections. **Synovium biopsy** is used to confirm cases that are especially difficult to diagnose. It requires insertion of an instrument called an arthroscope, used to remove synovium (joint lining) tissue.

Hemachromatosis is an inherited condition characterized by excess iron in the blood. This overabundance of iron exacerbates the damaging excess of free oxygen radicals generated by arthritis—especially the autoimmune activity in rheumatic diseases. In turn, free radicals promote inflammation and tissue damage. In this way, hemachromatosis considerably worsens damaging inflammations caused by arthritic diseases. In 1996, the National Institutes of Health began recommending that persons afflicted by arthritic inflammations be tested for hemachromatosis, which may be more common than once thought. Interestingly, the best remedy is performance of a good deed: the NIH identifies regular donation of blood as the best means of reducing the excess "iron load" produced by hemachromatosis.

Last, **X rays** are surprisingly unhelpful in detecting rheumatoid arthritis, as joints may not show any sign of wear in the early stages of the disease, despite significant pain. But X rays can help eliminate other problems such as stress injuries to joint tissues and bone.

PROGNOSIS OF RHEUMATOID ARTHRITIS

Rheumatoid arthritis can take one of several courses. It usually develops gradually, waxing and waning in intensity. Some patients experience a very sudden onset of severe symptoms. Cruelly, some enjoy what seems like a permanent remission, only to have full-blown symptoms return for several more years. The good news is that the inflammatory fires of rheumatoid arthritis often "burn out" with time. In fact, about one in ten patients returns to health within a year, and about half have complete remissions within two years. Like these short-term cases, many people who suffer rheumatoid arthritis later in life have relatively mild symptoms. Unfortunately, about 40% of rheumatoid arthritis patients experience harsher symptoms for six to eight years and are at high risk of suffering serious damage to their joints as well as osteoporosis (brittle bones). A key goal of treatment is to control the inflammations that initiate much of the tissue damage.

THE DANGER OF JOINT DAMAGE

The very real risk of suffering crippling joint damage places patients under great pressure to comply with standard drug treatments. They are often told to choose between compliance and joint destruction, but leading rheumatology researchers assert that this choice is a false one. In fact, no antirheumatic drug has been proved to prevent joint damage better over the long term than alternative pharmaceutical or natural drugs. Patients should not be frightened into blind obedience to medical orthodoxy. The fact is that patients respond differently to various drugs and other therapies. If all else fails, it may become necessary to try synthetic drugs, as indicated in Chapters 8 and 9. This is a choice between two evils—the risk of permanent tissue damage versus the uncertain benefits with potentially serious side effects.

PROGRESSION OF RHEUMATOID ARTHRITIS

The external symptoms associated with rheumatic diseases, as outlined here, are well known, but it is also important to understand what is going on inside affected tissues. The picture we will paint is based on research into rheumatoid arthritis, but much of it applies to other rheumatic diseases—except ankylosing spondylitis. Three things take place in joints affected by rheumatic diseases.

- **Autoimmune response:** Immune cells attack molecules in collagen or other joint tissues, probably because they mistake them for antigens (foreign substances).
- **Inflammation:** The first immune cell attack attracts other immune cells, which collect in the synovial membrane and begin to produce inflammatory chemicals. Synovial membrane cells also contribute inflammatory chemicals to the autoimmunity "fire."
- **Tissue destruction:** Synovial membrane cells grow in size and numbers, causing the membrane to thicken, deform, and expand. In some cases, the synovial membrane issues a granular tissue that grows right over the cartilage and subchondral bone. This overgrowth, called "pannus," releases enzymes called "collagenase," which degrade cartilage and bone. Inflammatory mediators in the synovial membrane absorb calcium from subchondral bone, causing further damage. Repeated inflammations in the joints disrupt the chemical processes that renew PGs—the major building blocks of cartilage. Together with the enzymatic destruction of collagen, this metabolic disruption leads to the joint damage that produces secondary osteoarthrosis.

INFLAMMATION:
WHY ARTHRITIC TISSUES CATCH FIRE

Chronic, fluctuating inflammations are the hallmark of rheumatoid diseases. Inflammation is beneficial under certain circumstances, because it plays important roles in aiding the body's immune response. For example, it increases blood flow to the affected region, thereby delivering needed nutrients, oxygen, and immune cells to an injured or infected area; speeding removal of dead bacteria and toxic bacterial secretions; and giving the area time to rest and heal by making it stiff and painful to move.

Unfortunately, the autoimmune attacks that characterize rheumatic diseases keep the inflammation response alive in the absence of any apparent outside threat to the body, making inflammation the chief source of tissue damage and pain. (The threat may be real but less damaging than the body's overreaction to it—see Chapter 14.) Since many of the rheumatic remedies discussed in Chapters 8 through 14 act by interrupting the course of chronic inflammation, it will be helpful to review the ways in which this key part of the human immune response is controlled by immune cells.

INFLAMMATORY MEDIATORS IN RHEUMATIC DISEASE

Immune cells initiate and control the inflammatory process in part by releasing messenger proteins called cytokines (e.g., interferons and tumor necrosis factors), which act like distress signals to all relevant immune cells. Specifically, cytokines tell other immune cells to initiate "cascade" reactions that yield hormonelike chemicals called inflammatory mediators. In rheumatic diseases, the inflammatory mediators that immune cells release in response to cytokine "messages" include histamine, leukotrienes, and certain prostaglandins. These inflammatory mediators make small capillaries wider and "leakier," permitting more immune cells to flood the area, where they release free radicals and enzymes that dissolve connective tissues.

Normally, inflammation is an appropriate immune response to injury or infection. But rheumatic diseases are characterized by an ungovernable, ongoing inflammation. We know that when synovial fluid contains high levels of cytokines, collagen damage and the risk of arthritis are both increased—and the cells that send the first inflammatory messages, via release of cytokines, may be distant from joint tissues.[2] We also know that damage to the synovial capsule corresponds to abnormally low levels of antioxidant molecules, including certain enzymes. Furthermore, damage to collagen correlates with high levels of inflammatory messenger molecules in synovial fluid (e.g., tumor necrosis factor-alpha, interleukin-1).[3]

To make matters worse, inflammation tends to raise fluid pressure within the synovial capsule of affected joints. When that pressure exceeds the pumping force behind blood coming in from surrounding vessels, blood and oxygen cannot reach the chondrocytes (cartilage cells). Ironically, lack of oxygen actually increases damage from free oxygen radicals, producing oxidative stress on blood vessels and further cutting blood circulation from subchondral bone to chondrocytes.

FREE RADICALS STOKE THE FIRE

The unstable oxygen compounds called "free radicals" are essential to life and to normal immune response, but they play a destructive role in chronic rheumatic inflammations. In what can become a vicious cycle, free radicals stimulate production of inflammatory mediators, which tend to stimulate production of more free radicals, and so on. Even after immune system cells release anti-inflammatory mediators, free oxygen radicals can keep the flame burning for a time. In rheumatoid arthritis patients, whose blood levels of antioxidant enzymes (glutathione, superoxide dismutase, catalase) are abnormally low, free radicals are left relatively unchecked to do damage.[4] Some of the supplements, herbs, and nutraceuticals we will review in later chapters are helpful precisely because they possess the antioxidant power to neutralize free oxygen radicals.

New research suggests that antioxidant compounds that act on cytokines—cutting off the inflammatory command at the source—may be even more important than the antioxidants that act to scavenge the free radicals that local immune cells release at the behest of cytokine messengers. These include carotenoids, essential fatty acids, soy isoflavones, vitamin E, branched-chain amino acids, curcumin, lipoic acid, and phenolic flavones from such foods as green tea, rosemary, and grape seed extract (OPC)—some of which we will discuss in depth in Chapter 13.

WHAT CAUSES RHEUMATIC DISEASE?

It is impossible to pin down the cause of most cases of rheumatic disease. But in evaluating various therapeutic options with your medical practitioner, knowledge of the probable causes and contributing factors will help you make rational treatment decisions.

THE AUTOIMMUNITY FACTOR

It is not certain why this happens, but the antibodies and immune cells of people with rheumatoid arthritis and lupus attack elements of connective tissues as though they were foreign invaders or were harboring disease microbes.[5] Immunologists categorize this process as a type III hypersensitivity reaction. This reaction does not seem to occur in ankylosing spondylitis (AS), which may not be an autoimmune disorder as they are normally understood. There are indications, however, that AS may be triggered by overgrowth of a bacteria that bears a close resemblance to certain tissues known to be present in AS patients (see "The Genetic Factor" in this chapter).

IMMUNE COMPLEXES AND RHEUMATOID ARTHRITIS

Normally, the body can distinguish between its own tissues, which immunologists call "self," and all foreign substances (antigens). Certain immune cells generate proteins called antibodies, which attach to antigens, hinder their activities, and mark them for destruction by immune cells. These antigen–antibody pairs are called "immune complexes." The inflammatory symptoms of rheumatoid arthritis usually wax and wane in tandem with the fluctuating levels of immune complexes in affected joints. The antigens in these immune complexes may arise from one or more of the three suspected causes of autoimmunity discussed later in this chapter: microbes, outlaw immune cells, and leaky gut syndrome. Each one may be responsible for a certain percentage of cases of rheumatoid arthritis and other rheumatic diseases, and any of them may be caused or exacerbated by the existence of a genetic predisposition to malfunctions in immune cells.

THE GENETIC FACTOR

Almost every cell in the body bears an "identification card" on its surface in the form of a marker molecule called HLA (human leukocyte antigen). Immune cells scan every cell they encounter, looking for HLA markers that differentiate body cells from invading disease microbes. But many people with rheumatic diseases have unusual types of HLA markers—either HLA-B27 or HLA-DR4, depending on the disease. These flawed HLA markers may lead immune cells to mount misguided attacks on the body's own tissues. The statistical evidence for a genetic factor in rheumatic diseases is compelling.

Rheumatoid arthritis: Two-thirds to three-quarters of people with rheumatoid arthritis have the HLA-DR4 marker as opposed to only one-quarter of the general population.

Ankylosing spondylitis: About 8% of the general population has the HLA-B27 marker, but almost all people with ankylosing spondylitis (90%) have it. And ankylosing spondylitis develops in 20% of all people with the HLA-B27 marker. British researchers found that peak periods of inflammation in ankylosing spondylitis coincide with peak levels of pathogenic *Klebsiella* bacteria. Abnormally high levels of *Klebsiella* organisms are an indicator of *dysbiosis*—the medical term for overgrowth of unfriendly bacteria in the intestines and colon.[6] On average, men have much higher *Klebsiella* counts and three times the risk of ankylosing spondylitis. This fact becomes even more intriguing when you consider that *Klebsiella* is the bacteria most similar to tissue with the HLA-B27 marker.

Reiter's syndrome: Of people with Reiter's syndrome, 63–96% possess the HLA-B27 marker and manifest signs of the disease after exposure to a sexually or intestinally transmitted microbe (e.g., *Chlamydia, Shigella, Salmonella, Yersinia, Campylobacter*).

Lyme disease: People who experience rheumatic joint symptoms from Lyme disease infection are more likely to have the HLA-DR4 marker. These genetic markers appear to make people susceptible to rheumatic diseases, but they do not seem to trigger them. For example, one in four people with HLA-DR4 markers never show signs of rheumatoid arthritis, and it is rare for both siblings in a pair of identical twins to have the disease.

One British study further supports the idea that people with flawed HLA markers must be exposed to some other stimulus in order to experience symptoms of rheumatic disease. Researchers examined seventeen families with more than one rheumatoid arthritis patient; compared with the general population, there was a slightly higher probability that additional family members would manifest the disease. There was also a smaller increase in the rate of rheumatoid arthritis among people who lived in the same households but had no blood relationship. This finding indicates that part of the higher risk among relatives may be due to environmental factors, such as pollution, infection, diet, or stress.[7]

SEX HORMONES

Some researchers have speculated that abnormally low levels of male or female sex hormones may lead to a higher risk of rheumatoid arthritis. This theory was put to the test in a clinical trial of 185 postmenopausal women with rheumatoid arthritis and a control group of 518 postmenopausal women free of disease. Among other factors, the authors measured levels of the master hormone DHEA (dehydroepiandrosterone) and the female hormone estradiol. Levels of DHEA were below normal in 86% of the arthritis patients and especially low among thirty-nine who were taking corticosteroids. There was no significant difference in the levels of estradiol found in the test and control groups.[8]

This study did not determine whether low levels of DHEA promote rheumatoid arthritis or result from it. Nevertheless, it seems reasonable for female patients to test the therapeutic effects of DHEA—especially in difficult cases. But caution is in order. Given the powerful and still mysterious effects of hormones, this decision should be made in consultation with a medical doctor or licensed naturopathic physician with your overall health status in mind.

SUSPECTED TRIGGERS OF RHEUMATIC DISEASE

Any of several suspected triggers are believed to be capable of causing rheumatic disease, especially in people possessing faulty HLA markers.

Immune Complexes

A variety of factors, including infections, leaky gut syndrome, or unknown causes, can lead to a buildup of immune complexes in joints. The immune cells' attempts to eliminate these immune complexes can damage surrounding joint tissues and may expose interior tissues, such as collagen, that are normally hidden from immune cells. Immune cells perceive these "sequestered" interior tissues as foreign invaders. Once exposed, sequestered tissues will elicit an autoimmune response that includes production of inflammatory mediators and cartilage-dissolving enzymes (collagenase).

Microbes

Throughout the first half of the twentieth century, most researchers believed that the autoimmune attacks on cartilage seen in rheumatic diseases were really attacks on microbes hiding in connective tissues. The chief suspects were viruses, streptococci bacteria, the tuberculosis bacillus, and, above all, a group of elusive microbes called *Mycoplasma* organisms. Today, an increasing body of evidence and more and more rheumatologists support this theory. For a more complete discussion of microbe theory and related antibiotic therapy, turn to Chapter 14.

Outlaw Immune Cells

Autoimmunity is puzzling, because immune cells are supposed to be programmed to distinguish between body tissues and foreign substances such as bacteria. Dramatic new findings from three American research teams suggest, however, that immune cells may not always rely on their internal programming to differentiate between self (body tissues) and antigens. Instead, immune cells may also rely on chemical signals from other immune cells to differentiate self from antigen.[9-11] If the immune cell issuing the signal to attack has mistaken self tissues for an antigen, the result can be sustained autoimmune attacks on the target tissues.

There is even a type of defective immune cell—known as a "self-reactive" T cell—that is capable of triggering misguided attacks on self tissues. The body sends newly made T cells—the "officer class" of the immune system—to the thymus gland, where they are programmed to distinguish body tissues from invaders. Some of the T cells never get these instructions and become self-reactive. A few of these defective T cells will make their way into the bloodstream. When the self-reactive T cells come near an inflamed organ or joint, they will drive through blood vessel walls, attack local tissues, and release chemical signals that prompt other immune cells to join in the attack. Other T cells, called suppressor cells, are supposed to intervene in such situations and call off the attack. But this cease-fire order may not work. The result can be a continuing autoimmune assault, even though the original inflammation was in tissues that normal T cells are programmed to recognize as self.

Leaky Gut Syndrome

This condition occurs when the spaces between cells in the intestinal walls become too big, usually the result of a food allergy, bacterial overgrowth, drugs (NSAIDs, steroids, antibiotics, etc.), or an intestinal inflammation. Leaky gut syndrome is believed to trigger ankylosing spondylitis in people with the HLA-B27 marker. It is also a suspected trigger of psoriatic arthritis and may be able to trigger rheumatoid arthritis. In fact, about two-thirds of all rheumatoid arthritis patients show signs of inflamed intestinal tissues.[12]

A leaky gut will permit large molecules, including bacterial toxins or incompletely digested foods, to pass into the bloodstream. Antibodies will treat them as antigens and attach to them, creating immune complexes. Some of the antigen molecules in these immune complexes can be chemically similar to proteins in joint tissue (e.g., collagen proteins). Because immune cells communicate with each other through the bloodstream, this resemblance may produce a "cross-reaction," in which immune cells begin to attack similar molecules in joint tissues.[13, 14] Even when it is not the cause of a rheumatic disease, leaky gut syndrome can aggravate symptoms by continuously introducing antigens into the bloodstream. Dietary changes can ameliorate this situation. The role of diet in treating rheumatic diseases is reviewed in Chapter 10.

Dysbiosis

Overgrowth of unfriendly bacteria and/or yeasts in the intestines—the condition known as dysbiosis—is often overlooked as a potential trigger of rheumatic disease. As seen in the case of ankylosing spondylitis (see "The Genetic Factor"), certain pathogens bear strong resemblances to the HLA markers associated with specific rheumatic diseases. If there is an overgrowth stemming from poor diet or extended courses of antibiotic therapy, the body may begin attacking its own tissues, mistaking them for pathogens with similar characteristics.

As with the close connection between AS and *Klebsiella*, British researchers found a strong association between HLA-DR4—the human leukocyte antigen found in two-thirds to three-quarters of people with rheumatoid arthritis—and the *Proteus* bacteria that are frequently responsible for chronic urinary tract infections.[15] Compared with men, women suffer much higher rates of both urinary tract infections and rheumatoid arthritis—another intriguing clue that points toward dysbiosis as a possible cause of rheumatic disease in persons with the "wrong" HLA markers.

FIBROMYALGIA: A SPECIAL CASE

We have included fibromyalgia syndrome (FMS) in this chapter because it shows signs of being an autoimmune disorder, albeit one that is not characterized by inflammation or detectable damage to connective tissues. Fibromyalgia is often thought of as a new disease and sometimes dismissed as a "fad" diagnosis. In fact, the Mayo Clinic produced an early description of the syndrome in 1943. The disease can be erroneously dismissed as a figment of patients' imaginations, because it has confusingly vague and diverse symptoms. Fibromyalgia affects about 3.5 million Americans, including 7% of persons more than 70 years of age, and is seven times more common among women than men. It is more common among people over the age of 50, and the statistical risk increases with age.

CAUSES

Some researchers believe that the symptoms of FMS are initiated by an injury to a specific area of tissue, whose effects somehow spread to other areas. However, about 50% of all fibromyalgia patients show previous symptoms of irritable bowel syndrome, and many show signs of other metabolic disorders (see "The Holistic Approach to Treatment"). There is also considerable evidence of autoimmunity. First, FMS is often associated with autoimmune disorders like rheumatoid arthritis (7% of FMS cases), Raynaud's syndrome (24%), and hyperthyroidism.[16] The immune dysfunction known as chronic fatigue syndrome (CFS) produces the numerous tender spots that typify FMS. In addition, anticardiolipin antibody has been found when FMS patients exhibit neuropathic symptoms, and the non-restorative sleep disorder seen in many patients with FMS are known to produce abnormalities in the immune system—including elevated levels of cytokines (e.g., interleukin-2).[17, 18]

SYMPTOMS AND PROGRESSION

According to 1990 classification criteria issued by the American College of Rheumatology, a diagnosis of fibromyalgia requires chronic muscular pain in at least eleven of eighteen common trigger points in contracted or tender areas of muscles, tendons, and ligaments. Typically, these trigger points are symmetrically located on both sides of the upper and lower body, usually at the knees, elbows, upper chest, and back and/or hips. The pain is in the muscles and their connecting tissues rather than inside joints. In addition, localized symptoms often include tingling sensations and muscle twitches. Like CFS, fibromyalgia is also associated with a broad range of seemingly unrelated symptoms, including fatigue, headaches, irritable bowel syndrome, depression, poor memory, fluid retention, insomnia, irritable bladder, premenstrual syndrome, and dizziness. Insomnia and nonrefreshing sleep are the single most common symptoms, characterized by an alpha-wave EEG, non-REM sleep abnormality. Also like CFS, there has been a long delay in the acceptance of fibromyalgia as a "real" rather than a purely psychosomatic disorder.

It appears that fibromyalgia's painful trigger points are centered on areas of ischemic (blood- and oxygen-deprived) muscle tissue. These trigger points may be produced by local injuries. Physical trauma to muscles can draw an increased volume of nerve impulses that will eventually make the affected tissues chronically oversensitized, contracted, and painful. Left untreated, fibromyalgia can worsen and even become physically or psychologically disabling. Holistic treatment of symptoms and possible underlying factors can lead to strong, lasting improvement but may not eliminate symptoms entirely.

PAIN MANAGEMENT

The first line of treatment is physical in nature and usually includes special exercises, application of heat, and physical or autogenic therapies. To be safe and effective, exercise should adhere to the guidelines set out by the National Fibromyalgia Research Association (see Appendix A). Treatments that restore circulation to ischemic tissues (neuromuscular therapy, shiatsu, etc.) may be beneficial, but they have not yet been subjected to clinical tests. In clinical trials, standard NSAIDs have proved no better than placebos in relieving fibromyalgic pain, but an experimental, opium-derived analgesic called tramadol hydrochloride has shown promise. And some patients gain months of relief at specific areas of pain following injection of anesthetic into the relevant trigger point.

TREATING DEPRESSION

Fibromyalgia can lead to depression, and it is important that it be dealt with immediately. Cognitive therapy can be very effective and should be tried. Doctors have also prescribed antidepressant drugs such as amitriptyline, with apparent benefit. Given the known side effects and risks of synthetic antidepressant drugs, it makes sense to first try well-researched herbs with similar effects, such as St. John's wort, kava, valerian, hops, and passionflower. Depression can quickly become a very serious condition; experiments with unproven treatments should be made under qualified medical supervision.

THE HOLISTIC
APPROACH TO TREATMENT

Physicians who approach fibromyalgia from a holistic perspective find that many patients show evidence of other causative or contributing factors, including food or chemical sensitivities, leaky gut syndrome, yeast (*Candida albicans*) infections, nutritional deficiencies, and impaired liver detoxification or digestive function. These doctors claim that treatment of these conditions typically produces improvement in fibromyalgia symptoms as well.

Holistic treatment also addresses metabolic deficiencies at the cellular level. All of the anti-inflammatory and immune-modulating nutrients, herbs, and nutraceuticals discussed in Chapters 11, 12, and 13 are of potential value. Supplements that promote restful sleep have shown benefit—especially 5-hydroxytryptophan, which the body uses to make the mood-elevating, relaxing neurotransmitter serotonin.[19]

Standard texts recommend NSAIDs to control pain, but these drugs promote leaky gut syndrome and the allergic reactions that appear to cause or exacerbate rheumatic conditions. Holistically oriented physicians instead recommend nutritional supplements that promote normal sleep and alleviate pain and anxiety, such as L-tyrosine, D,L-phenylalanine, gammahydroxybutyrate (GHB), 5-hydroxytryptophan, and, in combination, the amino acids L-arginine and L-orthinine.

Fibromyalgia patients show evidence of damage to the energy-producing centers (mitochondria) in their muscle cells, and they often suffer from low levels of magnesium and malic acid, both of which are critical to energy production. One small uncontrolled clinical trial found significant alleviation of pain and tenderness in twenty-four patients who received magnesium (200 milligrams) and malic acid (50 milligrams) over a six-month period.[20] Some patients also have low levels of the adrenal hormone DHEA. Anecdotal reports from physicians indicate that supplemental DHEA can boost energy levels and the ability to exercise. About one-third of fibromyalgia patients also have low levels of growth hormone, whose release may be stimulated by taking supplemental amounts of L-arginine and L-orthinine.

AN OVERVIEW OF RHEUMATIC DISEASES

CAUSATIVE FACTORS AND PAIN MANAGEMENT: AN ANALYSIS FROM THE FUNCTIONAL PERSPECTIVE

BY LEONID GORDIN, M.D.

IN THIS CHAPTER, I WILL REVIEW SEVERAL functional factors underlying the rheumatic diseases, which we explore more deeply in Chapters 6 (Rheumatic Diseases), 10 (Dietary Therapy), and 14 (Antibiotic Therapy). In addition, I will discuss pain and pain therapy from my perspective as a clinician treating patients for chronic pain. Conventional medicine has had relatively little success in curing rheumatic diseases or understanding their origins—perhaps because it has tended to focus on alleviation of symptoms with potent anti-inflammatory or immunity-suppressing drugs. Today most physicians agree that these multifaceted diseases demand a more sophisticated understanding of causes and contributing factors—an approach some have called "functional" medicine.

Functional medicine is a new approach to chronic, multifaceted conditions like rheumatoid arthritis, asthma, diabetes, and cardiovascular disease. In many cases, new evidence links these diseases to previously undetected factors like genetics or bacterial infection and to imbalances in the system, including such phenomena as leaky gut syndrome and excess free radicals. Increasingly, physicians and researchers are adopting a functional perspective, looking beyond symptoms and pathology to ask how chronic diseases are caused and why they are perpetuated.

While most chronic diseases have underlying genetic components, many individual cases appear to be triggered by negative lifestyle factors, such as lack of exercise or poor diet. Others can even stem from conventional medical treatments. For example, in the case of an acute injury, whether from physical trauma, infection, or toxins, the body is trying to contain and heal the condition. Sometimes this takes longer or causes more discomfort than we like. The usual medical response is to suppress symptoms with powerful drugs. Potent synthetic drugs can be indispensable in emergencies and valuable in certain chronic conditions, but they can disrupt the body's natural healing process and transform the problem into a chronic disease.

For instance, poor, low-fiber diets and excessive use of antibiotics or anti-inflammatory drugs can bring about leaky gut syndrome and dysbiosis (an unhealthy ratio of pathogens to beneficial bacteria in the intestines). Dysbiosis causes the body's metabolism and immune system to become weak and unbalanced. In other words, errors of omission or commission on the part of patients and physicians can turn acute conditions into serious, chronic conditions.

Given the preponderance of persuasive evidence for multiple, interacting causes, current research clearly supports a functional approach to the rheumatic diseases. Accordingly, my approach to treatment seeks to address root causes, while helping patients manage painful, destructive symptoms with the least toxic therapies.

FACTORS IN RHEUMATOID ARTHRITIS

When considering any chronic disease, we need to look to underlying causes or contributing factors, such as diet, nutrition, toxic drugs, and emotional stress. We consider treatment methods to stimulate the body's own healing powers, such as acupuncture, relaxation, and herbs. This approach allows the healing process to run a more natural course and avoids the problems related to potent drugs. A physician's first duty is to treat the pain and debilitation that brings a patient into the office. But the doctor must address the likely underlying causes—and any perpetuating behaviors or therapies—at the same time.

LEAKY GUT SYNDROME

Rheumatoid arthritis is considered an autoimmune disease—that is, one in which the body attacks its own tissues. What causes this dysfunction? There are certain suspicious functional factors we see in patients with rheumatoid arthritis. More than half show some evidence of leaky gut syndrome, which arises when there are gaps between the enterocytes—cells that constitute the intestinal walls. In leaky gut syndrome, large molecules can escape through the wall of the gut and into the bloodstream. When they are detected by the immune system, its B cells issue defensive proteins called antibodies, which lock onto the antigens (foreign substances) to mark them for destruction by other immune cells. We call the paired antigen and antibody an "immune complex."

In rheumatoid arthritis, immune complexes accumulate in the synovial fluid and around the cartilage. In some cases, antigens can resemble molecules in connective tissues, which fools the immune cells into attacking similar proteins in connective tissues. This probably occurs only in the presence of a predisposing factor, such as genetic flaws in the immune system, metabolic imbalance, chronic infection, food allergy, or drugs that promote leaky gut (NSAIDs, corticosteroids, antibiotics, etc.).

Rheumatoid arthritis may also be caused by deficiencies in the body's two-stage detoxification system. The overgrowth of disease bacteria associated with leaky gut syndrome—which medical science calls dysbiosis—results in a buildup of bacterial toxins. These pathogens release chemicals that suppress phase I liver detoxification. Deficiencies in phase II liver detoxification may be a factor as well. We know that people with rheumatoid arthritis are often deficient in sulfur, which is needed to make specific amino acids critical to this second stage of detoxification. If the detoxification system is not working well, antigens from a leaky gut can more easily find their way out of the bloodstream and into joints.

It usually makes sense to run a urine test for leaky gut. The patient is given mannitol, which should be able to enter the blood and then the urine. The patient is also given lactulose, which should not be able to enter the blood. If there is a lot of lactulose in the urine, it indicates leaky gut. And if there is too little mannitol, it means that the enterocytes are inflamed and cannot transport this smaller polysaccharide compound into the bloodstream, as they normally do. If the diagnosis is confirmed, the diet must be changed to allow the intestines to heal. People should eat whole grains, beans, vegetables, fruits, and a little bit of fish or poultry. They should avoid milk products and meat.

DYSBIOSIS: BACTERIAL OVERGROWTH

Patients can also suffer from bacterial overgrowth in the small intestine, which can play a role in rheumatic disease. The symptoms, such as bloating, cramps, diarrhea, and bad breath, are too commonplace to draw much attention. Conventional diagnosis is made by inserting an endoscopy tube and taking a biopsy. I prefer to use a breath test for alteration of gases. The patient drinks lactulose; if there is bacterial overgrowth, excess hydrogen and methane will be present in the breath, produced by bacterial fermentation of the lactulose.

FREE RADICAL STRESS AND CARTILAGE DEGENERATION

The synovial lining of the joints is rich in phospholipids, which contain unsaturated fats. Joints affected by rheumatoid arthritis are full of free oxygen radicals that will alter these fats. This affects the receptors for calcium and magnesium, for example, which leads to metabolic upsets in the cartilage and then to degeneration. In Chapter 3, we discuss the many downsides to standard NSAIDs like aspirin, and in Chapters 10, 11, 12, and 13 we look at safer dietary, herbal, and nutraceutical approaches to damping painful, destructive inflammations.

ACUTE AND CHRONIC PAIN

There are two basic types of pain—acute and chronic—and each requires a different approach to treatment. Acute, or "fast," pain feels specific, localized, and definable. It travels through a-delta nerve fibers, which are coated with a myelin sheath that allows rapid transmission. Osteoarthrosis patients often experience this kind of pain.

Most of the pain in arthritis is chronic, or "slow," pain, which is controlled by the brain's limbic system. The limbic system is the center of instincts and emotions, which is why chronic pain has an emotional component. People respond to chronic pain in various ways, depending on their personalities. Some react with maladaptive behavior, becoming sedentary, depressed, dependent on others, and too reliant on pain medications. At one time, frontal lobotomies were performed to relieve chronic pain—patients still felt the pain, but they either did not care or did not focus on it as much—a rather extreme solution to say the least. Chronic pain is called slow pain because it travels primarily through nonmyelinated (uninsulated) nerve fibers, making it slower to manifest as well as more diffuse and hard to pinpoint. Arthritis patients need to be aware that chronic pain can have a strong effect on their emotions.

PAIN MANAGEMENT

There are effective means of managing pain without overreliance on drugs. This does not imply any sort of moral or judgmental attitude toward analgesics. In cases of very serious, intractable pain, narcotics have unsurpassed analgesic effects and will not cause addiction. But such potent drugs are temporary methods of last resort. There are two viable nonpharmaceutical approaches to pain therapy. Each has its place and will work better in some people and circumstances than in others.

Cognitive therapy is a conscious effort to change one's attitude (see Chapter 2). It can be viewed as a sort of self-directed thought control, capable of changing old ways of thinking and feeling about things, including pain. Cognitive therapy is most effective when directed and supported by a trained therapist.

Autogenic training is a term that covers all the techniques designed to gain control over one's mental and nerve functions. Autogenic training includes such techniques as biofeedback, self-hypnosis, meditation, guided imagery, and progressive muscle relaxation. These techniques can produce measurable changes in skin temperature, electrical activity in muscles, and brain waves. One interesting biofeedback therapy helps patients gain control over tightness and pain in muscles through use of an electromyograph machine, which provides a readout of electrical activity in muscles.

Relaxation is the original, instinctive form of autogenic training.

Among other effects, it produces desirable changes in brain waves and causes release of endorphins, which are endogenous (internally produced) chemicals with analgesic, mood-lifting effects. There are many techniques for inducing relaxation, including meditation and biofeedback. It is important to learn how to let go of negative thoughts and feelings about pain, which is not the same as adopting a fatalistic attitude. With assistance from trained medical personnel, people can learn to control pain instead of letting it control them.

CHAPTER 7

GETTING THE RIGHT MEDICAL HELP

ALL RHEUMATIC DISEASES ARE SERIOUS conditions with the potential to turn lives upside down. In some cases, they can be crippling or even fatal. People suffering symptoms need to know what they are really facing before they can start dealing with it. Attempts to treat arthritic symptoms alone or with ill-informed medical guidance can result in otherwise preventable pain, impairment, and disability.

It is smart to assemble a medical team that offers expertise in every kind of treatment, including drugs, herbs, dietary supplements, and physical and mental therapies. A medical "team leader" who can help you assemble the group of practitioners best suited to your condition can be found among several categories of healers. The ideal may be a reputable holistic medical clinic that offers the best of conventional medicine and complementary natural methods.

RHEUMATOLOGISTS

If you suspect you have rheumatoid arthritis or a related rheumatic disease, the first person you should see is your primary physician.

Then you should consult a rheumatologist—a specialist who received up to five years of additional medical training in diagnosing and treating rheumatic diseases. Their services often cost more than a general practitioner's, but a good rheumatologist can be of great value even if you end up declining the drugs they recommend. Look for a rheumatologist readily willing to offer advice and monitor your condition during the course of any treatments you decide to try, conventional or otherwise. Should safer natural therapies fail to help you sufficiently, rheumatologists are usually well qualified to prescribe and monitor conventional drug treatments for rheumatic diseases.

RHEUMATOLOGY NURSE PRACTITIONERS

A rheumatology nurse practitioner can be a viable, even superior, alternative for treatment of rheumatoid arthritis diagnosed by a rheumatologist. One controlled study in Great Britain found that when compared with patients treated by rheumatologists, patients who were treated by nurse practitioners trained in rheumatology scored better on nine measures of effectiveness, including pain, joint mobility, and patients' own reports of satisfaction.[1] Much of the advantage was attributed to the fact that nurse practitioners were more likely to teach patients ways to minimize stiffness and improve mobility and refer patients for physical therapy, muscular massage, and so on.

OTHER MEDICAL DOCTORS

Rheumatologists are invaluable for diagnosing your condition and managing conventional drug therapy. But the world of rheumatology is a rather conservative specialty—perhaps in overreaction to the quackery that attaches to rheumatic diseases and other conditions that resist quick cures. What can you do if your rheumatologist ignores or downplays concerns you may have about conventional therapy or is reluctant to discuss other treatment options? If you cannot find a more open-minded rheumatologist, you can use another doctor as your medical team leader and consult him or her concerning the rheumatologist's advice. Your team leader should have significant experience treating rheumatic disorders, a thorough knowledge of your overall health condition, and a receptive attitude toward rational experimentation. Do not be shy about questioning a doctor's training and experience, because you cannot afford to risk misdiagnosis or inappropriate treatment.

HOLISTIC MEDICAL DOCTORS

Holistic medicine is both an attitude and an approach; it is not a peer-recognized, licensed specialty. Holistic physicians are grounded in science but acutely aware of the reality of bio-individuality and open to effective therapies wherever they may be found. Like naturopaths, holistic physicians draw on a more complete menu of medical options, including complementary therapies such as diet, nutrition, herbs, acupuncture, chiropractic, biofeedback, and stress reduction.

The multidimensional nature of rheumatoid arthritis calls for a holistic approach to treatment. To improve your chance of success while limiting the risk of side effects, look for a holistic doctor who offers three things: experience in treating your type of arthritis, familiarity with current research on rheumatic diseases, and experience using conventional and complementary therapies.

How will you know whether a doctor meets the last two criteria? It will be a good sign if he or she is familiar with the major theories and therapies covered in this book.

NATUROPATHS

The other type of specialist practitioner you should consider consulting is a naturopathic physician. Naturopathy also takes a holistic approach to medicine, based primarily on dietary, nutritional, and herbal therapies. Since the establishment of scientifically rigorous degree programs, it has become an increasingly respected offshoot of standard medicine. The naturopathic course of study encompasses key elements of a standard medical education—biochemistry, pharmacology, anatomy, physiology, pathology, among others—and a far more extensive education in complementary treatments, such as diet, nutritional supplements, and botanical medicines. If no one you know can recommend a competent, trustworthy naturopath, you can get in touch with graduates of the respected naturopathic colleges listed in Appendix A.

CHIROPRACTORS

Chiropractors specialize in manipulation of joints, nutritional therapy, and exercise therapy. When it comes to practicing complementary natural medicine, some chiropractors are top-drawer, with expertise comparable to that possessed by naturopaths. Given the variations in training and orientation among chiropractors, however, it is safer to rely on an experienced naturopathic physician or holistic doctor as your lead practitioner.

CHAPTER 8

CONVENTIONAL MEDICINES FOR RHEUMATIC DISEASES

CONVENTIONAL TREATMENTS FOR RHEUMATOID arthritis sometimes bring good, enduring results. But they often prove unsatisfactory, temporary, unhealthful, or intolerable. Leading rheumatologists recognize the problem. Dr. Wallace Epstein, Professor Emeritus of Medicine at the University of California, put the problem this way, in an article written in 1992 for fellow physicians: "No one really knows whether prednisone, gold injections, methotrexate, sulfasalazine, or hydroxychloroquine alter joint destruction and deformity associated with the disease. . . . Physicians . . . [prescribe these drugs] without solid evidence that they do more good than harm in the long run. Ten years after commencing treatment, virtually no rheumatoid arthritis patients still take these medications, either because they do not work, or because of side effects."[1]

Doctors divide treatments for rheumatic disorders into three broad categories. The NSAIDs, discussed in Chapter 3, are called "first line" drugs because they are often prescribed first. That is changing—many rheumatologists have come to favor earlier treatment with the so-called second-line drugs. The second-line drugs include disease-modifying antirheumatic drugs (DMARDs) and newer cytotoxic (cell-poisoning) drugs. Corticosteroids are in a third category all to themselves.

DISEASE-MODIFYING ANTIRHEUMATIC DRUGS (DMARDs)

There is considerable controversy, even among rheumatologists, concerning the value of DMARDs—a name that implies action on underlying mechanisms of the disease. In general, these chemicals seem to work by hindering attacks on connective tissue by immune cells. DMARDs can produce reasonably durable relief in a minority of cases, but they have several substantial shortcomings, specifically their toxic effects, limited benefits, and unknown risks. On average, DMARDs cause serious side effects, which are occasionally life threatening or irreversible, in at least 20% of patients. And although some patients do well on one or another DMARD for many years, their benefits are often of limited duration or scope. As one Scottish study found after following almost two hundred patients for five years, "Good control of disease activity and improved function can be achieved long term [five years] in approximately 30% of rheumatoid arthritis patients treated with injectable gold, sulfasalazine or penacillamine."[2] Lacking comparative research, it is not clear that DMARDs are better at lessening pain and stiffness than various combinations of safer therapies.

The totality of available evidence shows that 33–50% of patients taking DMARDs experience fair to excellent results for one to five years, with tolerable side effects or none at all. This means, however, that 50–67% experience side effects too severe to continue or gain only short-term or marginal relief. Patients are often prescribed the various DMARDs one after the other, as each fails or becomes intolerable. As one research team concluded, "There is no firm evidence that any of the commonly used drugs halted the progression of erosive disease."[3] Another team echoed this evaluation, saying: "[It is] a false assumption that short term clinical responsiveness equals long-term control."[4] As a rule, DMARDs have poorly understood effects—many significantly toxic—that may gradually undermine health.

AN AGGRESSIVE NEW STANCE ON DMARDs

Until recently, the standard treatment for rheumatoid arthritis and related diseases would begin with NSAIDs and work up to second-line drugs, on the theory that it is best to minimize use of the latter—for good reason, given their toxicity and limitations. Rheumatologists usually delayed use of DMARDs until joint damage was apparent. New radiographic evidence, however, shows that joint damage often occurs earlier than thought (within three years of diagnosis), and for this reason a more aggressive new approach has been widely adopted. Now patients are prescribed DMARDs virtually upon diagnosis. And because different drugs work on different aspects of the disease, it is more common for patients to be prescribed two or more drugs, including combinations of cortiocosteroids, cytotoxins, and DMARDs.

In 1996, *Annals of Internal Medicine* published the results of a study showing that patients who received early treatment with DMARDs had less disability, pain, and joint damage than patients taking only NSAIDs, but they also suffered more adverse effects. In August of 1997, *The Lancet* published the results of a trial testing a combination therapy consisting of a cortiocosteroid (prednisolone), a cytotoxin (methotrexate), and a DMARD (sulfasalazine). At the end of the seven-month trial, 72% of patients showed improvement versus only 49% of the controls, who took sulfasalazine alone. These are important results, but no one yet knows the long-term effects of this aggressive new approach.

GOLD

Modern drug treatment for rheumatoid arthritis began with the curious case of a drug that went from quackery to cure back to quackery, at last attaining its current status as a leading conventional therapy. Once the alchemists' Holy Grail, gold long reigned as the rheumatologist's hardy perennial. This controversial metallic medicine has become a standby drug despite the potential for serious side effects and a continuing lack of evidence for long-term effectiveness.[5] Injected gold salts have been used since the turn of the century, first as a tuberculosis drug. Gold became standard rheumatoid arthritis therapy in the 1920s, when the disease was widely thought to be infectious in origin—an idea that is staging a comeback, as described in Chapter 14.

Doubts about the germ theory of rheumatoid arthritis and awareness of the side effects from excessively aggressive use led to virtual abandonment of gold therapy through the 1940s. By the end of that decade, new studies had shown lower doses of gold salts to be effective while causing fewer, milder side effects. Until the advent of methotrexate (see "Methotrexate" in this chapter), gold was the unquestioned DMARD of choice for rheumatoid arthritis. It remains the first choice of rheumatologists concerned about the long-term toxicity of methotrexate, despite evidence that methotrexate is no more toxic than gold.

Gold administered in monthly injections provides very good pain relief in about one-third of all cases and delivers middling results in about one of five patients. It can take from several weeks to six months to know if gold is going to work. Gold therapy has side effects, including mouth sores, diarrhea, rashes, or itching in one of three patients. One in six patients suffers side effects (blood or organ toxicity) serious enough to force them to stop gold therapy. This is why regular monitoring and blood tests are required for patients taking it. Even when detected early, toxic damage to organs is not always reversible. A new study also shows that one form of injected gold (sodium thiomalate) can cause dizziness, nausea, and pain and may increase the risk of heart attacks and strokes.[6]

Oral gold is a new form that seems to be somewhat less effective, gives rise to diarrhea in many patients, and may be riskier in other ways. Since patients can take oral gold at home, they do not need to visit their doctor regularly and might miss the periodic blood tests needed to detect gold's dangerous toxic effects.

HYDROXYCHLOROQUINE

This antimalaria drug has been used against rheumatoid arthritis almost since its introduction in 1967. Like gold, it is usually very slow-acting, with about one-third of patients reporting good results.[7] Hydroxychloroquine is considered relatively safe, but it leads to intolerable gastric side effects and changes in skin color in one of five patients. Psychoneurological symptoms (seizures, nightmares, excitability) occur in rare cases. Like other quinine derivatives, hydroxychloroquine often causes temporary blurred vision, which is not considered a reason to stop taking it. In less than 1% of patients, hydroxychloroquine poses long-term use risks to vision, by damaging the retina. For this reason, patients on hydroxychloroquine must have an eye examination every three to six months.

PENICILLAMINE

Penicillamine, a synthetic offspring of penicillin, has been used against rheumatoid arthritis for more than thirty years. Before it was tried in rheumatoid arthritis, penicillamine was used to remove toxic metals from people poisoned by them. Penicillamine is most effective for two kinds of patients—those with the specific genetic marker HLA-DR2 and those unresponsive to other DMARDs.

The drug's many significant side effects, however, force two of five patients to abandon it within months, and 60% reject it within two years.[8] Those who are not forced to discontinue penicillamine report good results one-third of the time, and one-fifth report only minor relief. In addition to causing some of the same side effects as gold and hydroxychloroquine, penicillamine can lead to kidney or bone marrow damage, muscle weakness, and autoimmune disorders. Accordingly, patients must undergo regular blood and urine tests.

SULFASALAZINE

Like gold, sulfasalazine has had its ups and downs in rheumatology practice. It was developed just after the turn of the century by Swedish researchers who wished to combine the newly discovered antimicrobial properties of sulfur with the active ingredient in aspirin (salicylate). Like gold, this drug was developed because microbes were believed to be responsible for rheumatoid arthritis. It was thrown out of mainstream rheumatology in the 1940s, along with the microbial theory of rheumatoid arthritis. Subsequent research, however, has shown sulfasalazine to be quite effective and more so in combination with methotrexate. Many rheumatologists prescribe it despite lack of FDA approval for use in rheumatoid arthritis, which may be granted soon. The most common side effects are nausea (one of five cases), headaches, dizziness, urine crystals, allergic reaction, or rashes. In rare cases, sulfasalazine can produce serious blood and liver toxicity and temporary low sperm count.

ANTIBIOTICS

Like gold and sulfasalazine, antibiotics were originally used to treat rheumatoid arthritis in the belief that some as yet unidentified germ was causing the disease. And like gold and sulfasalazine, antibiotics have gone in and out of fashion for the past fifty years along with the changing winds of arthritis theory. Regardless of continuing uncertainty over the role of microbes in causing rheumatoid arthritis and its symptoms, new clinical evidence indicates that certain antibiotics may rival or exceed the efficacy of conventional rheumatoid arthritis drugs—with fewer, milder side effects.

The history of antibiotic therapy for rheumatic diseases, with its alternating periods of acceptance and rejection by mainstream medicine, offers an object lesson in the fickle, often unscientific nature of scientific consensus (see Chapter 14). The reemergence of microbe theory and antibiotic therapy may prove to be a turning point in the understanding of arthritis.

CYTOTOXIC DRUGS

Like DMARDs, cytotoxic drugs are believed to work by hindering the immune system in its attack on connective tissues. Cytotoxins are a bit different, in that they specialize in slowing the body's production of antibodies. The prefix *cyto-* means "cell," and each of these drugs was originally used either as chemotherapy to kill cancer cells or as a means of crippling the body's immune attack on transplanted organs. Cytotoxins work more quickly than DMARDs, but they are also more dangerous.

A representative tragedy that occurred in 1996 points up the risks of these potent drugs. Lorraine Hurley, a 67-year-old Massachusetts woman with rheumatoid arthritis, took her granddaughter to a fast-food restaurant. They and forty-two other patrons soon became ill from *Salmonella* bacteria in the food. All recovered quickly except Ms. Hurley, who fell into a coma and died nineteen days later. As the local newspaper reported, "Infectious disease specialists said yesterday that the food poisoning death of Lorraine Hurley was most likely brought on because her immune system was weakened by severe dehydration and . . . the immunosuppressant medication methotrexate [she was taking] for her rheumatoid arthritis."[9] According to the attending physician, Ms. Hurley might be alive today had she not been taking the drug, yet methotrexate is quickly becoming the most widely prescribed antirheumatic medicine.

METHOTREXATE

Developed in the 1940s as an anticancer chemotherapy drug, methotrexate is overtaking gold as the prime therapeutic choice of rheumatologists. The drug inhibits production of antibodies and in this way lowers the number of immune complexes in joints that are available to be attacked by immune cells. Methotrexate may also work by inhibiting folic acid, a B vitamin needed to reproduce cells, including immune cells implicated in the autoimmune attacks on rheumatic joints.[10] It is also possible that methotrexate blocks the inflammatory process after it is initiated by immune cells.[11] This medicine presents patients with hard choices, since the evidence for its efficacy and safety is very contradictory.

In its favor, methotrexate seems to relieve symptoms quite effectively in about half of those for whom it is prescribed, especially if taken within the first five years of disease onset. A number of studies suggest that methotrexate is effective and tolerable for up to 70% of patients for periods lasting as long as five years.[12, 13] One study that followed patients for a mean period of seven years found significant prevention of crippling joint erosion; other studies have not found as much benefit.[14, 15] Methotrexate has strong anti-inflammatory effects that relieve swelling and tenderness. And, except for antibiotics, methotrexate is the fastest-acting second-line drug, with its effects usually apparent within a month.

On the other hand, methotrexate use requires close monitoring, because the drug has serious side effects in a small but significant percentage of patients. It has been used as an anticancer therapy since the early 1950s, but usually for short periods of time at high doses. Far lower doses of methotrexate have been used for rheumatoid arthritis since 1988, and knowledge of the long-term side effects is limited. By the ten-year mark, less than 30% of patients still experience benefit without intolerable side effects.[16] In fact, a new study indicates that only 16% of patients taking methotrexate enjoy even a minor, 20% alleviation of symptoms (e.g., one-fifth fewer painful joints). Conversely, this means that 84% of the patients taking methotrexate experience even less abatement in symptoms.[17]

Methotrexate produces one or more side effects, ranging from mild to serious, in up to 90% of patients who take it.[18, 19] The majority of these effects, which include nausea, frequent infections, hair loss, inflamed intestinal walls, and diarrhea, can be cut down by lowering the dosage or making other changes in the therapeutic regimen. Methotrexate can also cause more serious side effects, including liver dysfunction, gastric ulcers, and bleeding, in 15–20% of patients. In rare cases (1–2%), it can lead to potentially fatal lung inflammation and liver scarring. To prevent these effects, blood tests are required every two to four weeks. This major inconvenience is given little weight in medical evaluations of methotrexate versus alternatives.

If you decide to try methotrexate, be aware that supplemental folic acid has been shown to lower the incidence of side effects. In one study, folic acid cut down the incidence of adverse effects from 89% of patients taking methotrexate alone to 48% of patients taking methotrexate plus 5 milligrams of folic acid per week. Do not take higher doses of folic acid, since they do not work as well.

OTHER CYTOTOXIC DRUGS

Four other immunity-suppressing cancer drugs can be used when patients prove unresponsive to methotrexate or DMARDs. These newer cytotoxins are cyclophosphamide, chlorambucil, azathioprine, and cyclosporine. About half of all patients who try these drugs experience at least temporary relief from one of them. But this relief is accompanied by serious side effects, including nausea, vomiting, hair loss, dangerously impaired immunity, and significant risk of infertility, liver or lung damage, and, in some cases, cancer.[20] Methotrexate has been shown to work better, with fewer side effects, when taken at lower doses with azothioprine or cyclosporine. There is one exception to this rule. Taking methotrexate with cyclosporine greatly increases the risk of an overgrowth of body hair.[21]

CORTICOSTEROIDS

It must have seemed a miracle to rheumatoid arthritis patients when corticosteroids were introduced in 1948—a feat that won the researchers twin Nobel Prizes two years later. Patients taking oral corticosteroids, such as cortisone and prednisone, experienced dramatic relief from inflammation and pain. Only later did the drugs' many serious side effects—most related to prolonged use—become apparent.

Corticosteroids are important hormones secreted by the adrenal gland, which regulates key metabolic functions. These drugs are the most dramatically effective anti-inflammatory substances known, but their benefits often bear a high price tag. Routine use can lead to serious side effects, including diabetes, stomach ulcers, weight gain, osteoporosis, thin skin, slow wound healing, muscle weakness, cataracts, insomnia, hypertension, susceptibility to infections, easy bruising, and psychological problems. Corticosteroids must be withdrawn from use gradually to avoid serious illness or even death. They may be injected in specific joints once every four to six months with little risk of adverse reactions. Doctors rarely prescribe them today, except to help patients through a period of severe symptoms while waiting for a DMARD to take effect.

A NEW APPROACH:
BIOLOGIC RESPONSE MODIFIERS

Improved understanding of the mechanisms of rheumatic inflammation has led to the development of potentially useful drugs, all of which are undergoing clinical trials and must be injected regularly. In the fall of 1997, the American College of Rheumatology heard presentations on three drugs under development. Each of these so-called biologic response modifiers interferes with messenger chemicals involved in inflammation. None is considered a cure or a full replacement for DMARDs, nor is any one of them capable of completely halting the destruction of joints. In each case, patients will need to take the drug for life, but, based on clinical results to date, these new biologic response modifiers may offer considerable long-term relief from rheumatic symptoms.

INTERLEUKIN-1 INHIBITORS

The biotech company Amgen is developing a drug that suppresses the activity of interleukin-1, the protein that induces inflammation by activating cells lining the blood vessels. Researchers at the University of Pittsburgh have also inserted bioengineered genes into rheumatic joints, stimulating production of a protein that dampens interleukin-1 activity. A small number of volunteers have benefited from this therapy.

MONOCLONAL ANTIBODIES

Pharmaceutical firms IDEC and Smith Kline Beecham are cooperating on production of a monoclonal antibody (drug-delivering protein) that works by binding to the surface of system T cells, slowing the autoimmune responses that these "command and control" cells inappropriately initiate and maintain in rheumatic diseases. Final Phase III clinical trials began in late 1997. (Phase III clinical trials are the last step needed to prove efficacy in the hope of genuine approval by the FDA.)

CYTOKINE INHIBITORS

Tumor necrosis factor (TNF) is a key cytokine (messenger protein) in rheumatic inflammations. At the end of 1997, Immunex Corp. began Phase III clinical trials of their injectable TNF drug. Called Enbrel, or TNFR:Fc, the drug is a receptor molecule that binds to TNF circulating in the blood. The results, published in July of 1997 in the *New England Journal of Medicine,* suggest that Enbrel is reasonably safe and effective, with remarkably few side effects. Among the participants who received the highest dose, Enbrel injections decreased the number of swollen joints by 20%; eased swelling by 61% (versus 25% of the placebo-injected group); and lessened pain and stiffness and improved quality of life in half of the participants. Some patients enjoyed a virtual cure during the first twelve months but later saw a return of symptoms in milder form.

Other research by Immunex shows that when they are taken together, Enbrel and methotrexate work better than methotrexate alone. To date, it remains unclear whether Enbrel can prevent joint damage. And the long-term effects beyond the fifteen-month duration of the trial are unknown. In May of 1998, Immunex applied to the FDA for approval to market Enbrel, and the company hopes to receive permission by the end of 1998.

Early in 1998, the FDA approved a similar drug, called Avakine, for use in Crohn's disease, an inflammatory autoimmune disorder of the intestines. (Unlike Enbrel, Avakine disrupts TNF binding to immune cells through the action of monoclonal antibodies.) The manufacturer, Centocor, Inc., of Malvern, Pennsylvania, is expected to file for approval for the use of Avakine in rheumatoid arthritis by mid-1999. At present, under current "off label" prescription rules, doctors can legally use the drug for any rheumatic condition.

TACE BLOCKERS

Early in 1997, Immunex Corp. announced discovery of an enzyme called TACE, which acts very early in the inflammation process by initiating release of TNF. Immunex is working on an oral form, to avoid the need for injections.

EXPERIMENTAL THERAPIES

Work is proceeding on a number of other fronts, including vaccinations, stem cell or bone marrow transplants, antibody blood filters, and genetic screening.

ALTERNATIVE OPTIONS

The dilemma facing patients in distress lies in deciding whether the alternatives have been exhausted and how long they can afford to wait for other measures to start working before serious joint damage occurs. This decision should be made with medical guidance. As we will see, there are realistic alternatives for protecting joints and relieving symptoms with a higher degree of safety.

CHAPTER 9

CONSUMER'S GUIDE TO RHEUMATIC REMEDIES

THE PURPOSE OF THIS BOOK IS TO provide reliable information that may help people make better informed therapeutic choices. The large number of options can be confusing and can force patients to fall back on conventional wisdom—a decision that may not always be wise. This chapter will help you prioritize the many choices covered in Chapters 8 through 16. Remember that the physical and psychological therapies discussed in Chapter 2 can be highly effective and should be considered indispensable adjuncts to herbal, nutraceutical, and pharmaceutical remedies.

USING THE REMEDIES TABLES

Each of the rheumatic remedies covered in this book was researched to determine (to the extent it is possible) the quality and quantity of the scientific and historical evidence for therapeutic claims. We then assigned each a ranking, based on our judgment of relative efficacy and safety.

PRIORITIZING WITHIN CATEGORIES

Remedies are presented in descending order (top to bottom) of recommended priority. The exceptions to this prioritization scheme are vitamins and minerals. While they are listed here in descending order of presumed efficacy (i.e., vitamin C is most important, then vitamin E, etc.), patients should take all of them every day. In fact, arthritis patients should take a multivitamin supplement that contains all of the essential vitamins and minerals every day. Our list is intended to help you prioritize purchase and use of supplemental doses of vitamins and minerals that offer the greatest therapeutic potential.

PRIORITIZING ACROSS CATEGORIES

The categories are prioritized from left to right in descending order of importance. Together, dietary therapy and vitamins and minerals are recommended as the first priority. It makes sense to try this purely nutritional regimen first, so that you will know whether it alone can relieve your symptoms and protect joints.

RANKING RHEUMATIC REMEDIES

Rheumatic remedies in the table are listed in rough order of efficacy, based on the limited data available to date. In other words, we recommend you try diet and vitamins first and then take the herbal and nutraceutical remedies, starting with the ones placed at the top of their respective lists and moving down the list as needed. Given the paucity of comparative studies, our judgments are necessarily subjective. Be sure to consult your physician, since circumstances vary and the most important goals are to support normal living and to prevent joint and organ damage. In devising the table of remedies, we kept the several overall rankings in mind.

TABLE OF REMEDIES

1ST PRIORITY (START WITH BOTH)		2ND PRIORITY	3RD PRIORITY
Diet (Chapter 10)	Vitamins/Minerals* (Chapter 11)	Herbs (Chapter 12)	Nutraceuticals (Chapter 13)
Seven- to fourteen-day liquid fast under medical supervision	Take each one daily in the doses listed in Chapter 11*	Take daily for pain and inflammation or as needed	Take daily for pain and inflammation or as needed
Follow up with a daily diet that favors unrefined plant foods and minimizes intake of potentially allergenic foods	Vitamin C	Boswellia	Take daily for pain and inflammation or as needed.
	Vitamin E	Ginger	Omega-3 essential fatty acids
	B vitamins	Shosaikoto (Chai' hu)	CMO
	Selenium	Devil's claw	OPC (grape seed extract)
	Boron	Lei-gong-teng	Curcumin
	Zinc	Secondary herbs	Enzymes
	Bovine cartilage	Capsaicin	Sea cucumber
	Green-lipped New Zealand mussel	Other herbs and Chinese patent medicines (listed in Appendix B)	Topical emu oil

* All of these can be obtained from a multivitamin/mineral supplement. Add more as needed to meet the doses suggested in Chapter 11.

If a rheumatologist determines that joint damage is not an immediate concern, give the combination of **diet, vitamins,** and **minerals** four to twelve weeks to work before trying other remedies. See Chapter 11 for suggested dosages, which in some cases are higher than in most multivitamin supplements. **Herbs** and **nutraceuticals** should be explored one at a time. Take each remedy for at least two weeks before judging the results. If symptoms are severe, you can try taking herbs and nutraceuticals in various combinations. For example, boswellia, ginger, curcumin, and OPC are comparably potent anti-inflammatory agents that may provide stronger relief when any two are taken together. COX-2 NSAIDs (Celebra, etc.) can be taken at any time to relieve pain, if herbs or nutraceuticals (ginger, curcumin) fail to provide sufficient relief.

Antibiotics are the logical next step should diet, vitamins, herbs, and nutraceuticals fail to halt pain and joint destruction. **Synthetic drugs** (DMARDs, cytotoxins, biologic response modifiers) are drugs of last resort, unless your condition shows no sign of improving or medical tests reveal signs of joint damage.

CHAPTER 10

DIETARY THERAPY IN RHEUMATIC DISEASES

A CONDITION CALLED LEAKY GUT SYNDROME is found in many people with rheumatic diseases. Research on multiple sclerosis—an inflammatory, autoimmune disease affecting connective nerve tissues—found that mortality is increased by diets high in saturated fats from meat and dairy foods and decreased by diets high in unsaturated fats from marine and plant foods.[1] In addition, Mediterranean diets high in plant foods and monounsaturated fats—that is, olive oil— inhibit expression of glycoproteins that trigger some of the adverse immune and inflammatory reactions characteristic of rheumatic diseases. In fact, a preponderance of laboratory and clinical research suggests that leaky gut syndrome, dysbiosis (intestinal overgrowth of pathogenic bacteria), and/or diets high in animal fats are triggering or aggravating factors in many cases of rheumatic disease.

LEAKY GUT SYNDROME

As we saw in Chapter 6, leaky gut syndrome—otherwise known as permeable bowel—may trigger the autoimmunity dysfunction that characterizes rheumatic diseases. Conversely, leaky gut can result from and aggravate autoimmunity (see Chapter 6). A permeable bowel allows incompletely digested foods to leak into the blood, producing an immune response believed to be capable of causing food allergies or autoimmunity. Leaky gut syndrome can be caused by chronic dysbiosis and extended use of antibiotics or NSAIDs, among other factors. Whether leaky gut is a cause or a result of autoimmunity, it is clear that dietary changes can relieve or even eliminate symptoms in some patients with rheumatic conditions.

STOMACH ACID (HYPOCHLORHYDRIA) AND RHEUMATIC DISEASE

There is also significant evidence that some rheumatoid arthritis patients do not secrete enough hydrochloric acid to fully digest their food—a condition known as hypochlorhydria.[2] Like leaky gut syndrome, this gastric acid deficiency can allow food particles to escape into the bloodstream, leading to an allergic reaction that can trigger or aggravate autoimmunity. Rheumatic patients should have a gastric acid analysis to test for hypochlorhydria. There is a remedy, in the form of hydrochloric acid/pepsin supplements.

THERAPEUTIC DIETS

There are ample theoretical grounds to suspect that there are connections among leaky gut syndrome, dysbiosis, food allergies, diets high in animal fats, and rheumatic diseases. Most doctors dismissed these links until the late 1980s and early 1990s, when the results of new research lent strong support to two theories.

- Fasting and vegetarian diets can limit the activity of immune cells and inflammatory mediators in joint tissues.
- Diets high in plant foods and/or low in suspected food allergens can lessen the severity of inflammatory rheumatic symptoms in many patients.

The clinical trials that produced these findings fell into three categories: studies of temporary fasting, studies of temporary fasting followed by plant-based diets, and studies of plant-based diets that are also low in suspected food allergens. The therapeutic diets these trials employed were designed to eliminate or decrease intake of animal and refined foods as well as suspected allergens—among them, milk products, gluten (in wheat, rye, barley, oats), and members of the nightshade botanical family, including potatoes, bell peppers, eggplant, and tomatoes.

EVIDENCE FOR FASTING

Based on the limited evidence collected to date, it appears that brief liquid fasts (one to two weeks) can bring temporary improvement. To quote the conclusions of one Swedish group, "Otherwise healthy and well-nourished patients with rheumatoid arthritis show significant clinical improvement from practicing prolonged fasting for 7 to 10 days. The improvement is reversible and lost when eating is taken up again. Although of little [long-term] therapeutic value, the anti-inflammatory effect of short-term fasting is of significant interest and better understanding of the mechanisms is desirable."[3]

In line with the results of other studies, another group of Swedish researchers found that the positive results were explained in part by related effects on the immune system and its inflammatory responses: "Its [fasting's] mechanisms are complex and involve diminished activation of neutrophils and lymphocytes [immune cells] and decreased generation of leukotrienes [key inflammatory mediators] and of concentration of serum complement factors [immune proteins], as well as of other proinflammatory systems. . . . Other metabolic and endocrine changes may be of significance. . . ."[4, 5] While it is not evidence for the positive effect of fasting, one study showed significant improvement in the symptoms of rheumatoid arthritis among female patients who adopted a low-fat diet.[6] However, authors of two more recent studies found hints that low-fat diets can be counterproductive. One group found that a low-fat diet reduced blood levels of vitamin E and increased pro-inflammatory prostaglandins,[7] and another found symptoms of rheumatoid arthritis were the worst among people lowest in body fat.[8]

EVIDENCE FOR PLANT-BASED DIETS

Several well-controlled clinical trials have tested the effects of an initial fast followed by a plant-based diet that is not exclusively vegetarian. In a landmark Norwegian study lasting a full year, fifty-three patients were randomly assigned to two groups of equal size. One-half were test subjects who went to a health farm. The rest, who ate a normal diet at a convalescent home, acted as a control group.

The test subjects at the health farm started with a seven- to ten-day liquid fast, followed by 3.5 months on a gluten-free vegetarian diet. Dairy products were gradually introduced over the remainder of the year. The results were dramatic, with the test subjects enjoying improvements in the number of tender or swollen joints, stiffness, grip strength, and all other clinical and laboratory measures of disease severity. The control group saw only a mild improvement in pain. As the researchers concluded, "The benefits in the diet group were still present after one year, and evaluation of the whole course showed significant advantages for the diet group in all measured indices. This dietary regimen seems to be a useful supplement to conventional medical treatment of rheumatoid arthritis." [9, 10]

EVIDENCE FOR
HYPOALLERGENIC DIETS

Other trials tested the theory that many rheumatoid arthritis patients are allergic to certain foods—allergies that may give rise to rheumatoid arthritis symptoms. In one well-regarded study, experienced British rheumatology researchers divided fifty-three subjects into two groups. Both groups were taken off their usual drugs and given placebo and acetaminophen pills for two weeks. Group 1 was put on a "hypoallergenic" diet free of suspected allergens for one week, after which possible food allergens (dairy, nightshade vegetables, gluten, etc.) were reintroduced one by one over a five-week period. When anyone in Group 1 seemed to react adversely to a food, it was withdrawn from that person's diet, producing a customized hypoallergenic diet for each person. During the same time period, the volunteers in Group 2 continued eating their regular diet and taking placebo and acetaminophen pills. After six weeks, Group 2 switched to the test diet and continued on it for six weeks.

In the end, both groups responded very well to the hypoallergenic diet. The researchers put it this way: "In a blind, placebo-controlled study of dietary manipulation therapy in outpatients with rheumatoid arthritis there was significant objective improvement during periods of dietary therapy compared with periods of placebo treatment, particularly among good responders. Possible explanations include reduced food intolerance [from identifying and eliminating allergenic foods], reduced gastrointestinal permeability [from stopping NSAIDs], and benefit from weight loss and from altered intake of substrates for prostaglandin production [arachidonic acid from animal fats]." [11, 12]

Two other clinical trials, one conducted in India and one in Holland, tested the effects of giving patients a diet free of dairy foods, gluten (allergenic protein fraction of grains), and meats. The researchers then measured the effects of reintroducing these foods one by one.[13, 14] Different patients reacted to different foods, with some being sensitive to many of the potential food allergens. The evidence that food allergies play a part in rheumatoid arthritis, however, is mixed. Another study in Norway compared the effects of a hypoallergenic diet versus a diet high in such suspected allergens as tomatoes, gluten, milk, meat, citrus, and peas. The patients on the hypoallergenic diet enjoyed a decrease in the number of tender joints, but overall the results were not very significant.[15]

A well-controlled, ten-week U.S. study investigating the effects of an "anti-arthritis" vegetarian diet promoted in a popular book found little difference between test subjects and controls. Two of the test patients, however, improved so much that they stayed on the diet and reported relapses whenever they abandoned it. The researchers' conclusions, reached before the positive studies described earlier were published, represent a conservative evaluation of the evidence for dietary therapy: "Our study failed to provide evidence of objective overall clinical benefit. . . . However, our data are not inconsistent with the possibility that individualized dietary manipulations might be beneficial for selected patients with rheumatic diseases."[16] We should note that one study found no association between symptom-aggravating foods, as reported by rheumatoid arthritis patients, and the results of standard blood tests to identify food allergens.[17]

IS BELIEF A FACTOR IN DIETARY THERAPY?

The Norwegian investigators whose health farm study showed dramatic success found that patients' personal psychology and attitude may also play a role. Compared with a random group of rheumatoid arthritis patients, the test subjects whose symptoms had improved during a one-year clinical test of fasting and vegetarian diets possessed certain psychological factors in common—greater self-reliance, a distrust of the medical establishment, and more faith in alternative treatments. They also found that their experimental vegetarian diet reduced stress, which is believed to affect the severity of symptoms.

ORAL TOLERANCE THERAPY

Some of the most intriguing clues that arthritis is connected to leaky gut syndrome and food allergies come from therapeutic successes with oral tolerance therapy. This experimental treatment is closely related to desensitization therapy, where hay fever sufferers are treated with increasingly potent administrations of pollen, dust, and other allergens. This gradually decreases their immune systems' overreaction to harmless airborne substances.

Inspired by this example, researchers have attempted to halt the autoimmune attacks of rheumatoid arthritis in a similar fashion. The assumption researchers made was that rheumatoid arthritis may be caused by dietary collagen slipping into the blood from a leaky gut. They tested this theory by asking volunteers to consume small amounts of sterilized chicken collagen. Strong preliminary successes with this therapy support the idea that leaky gut syndrome is a possible trigger for rheumatoid arthritis. It is a case of reverse logic along the following lines. Collagen molecules in dietary meats and poultry are attacked as foreign invaders when they leak into the bloodstream. This response may trigger autoimmunity attacks on the body's collagen-rich connective tissues, producing rheumatic disease. Researchers theorized that if the immune system were carefully reintroduced to collagen as a harmless food in the gut rather than as a foreign body (antigen) in the blood, special immune suppresser cells would command other immune cells to treat the body's own collagen as friendly material.[18, 19]

So far the results have been mixed. In one clinical study, patients with severe, active rheumatoid arthritis experienced significant relief after ingesting specially prepared chicken collagen; several enjoyed a total, enduring remission.[20] Commercial oral tolerance drugs developed at Harvard Medical School, however, scored little better than a placebo in FDA-approved clinical trials. Colloral, developed for rheumatoid arthritis, and Myloral, for multiple sclerosis, failed to outperform placebos, but the results achieved with higher doses of Colloral (60 micrograms per day) in selected patients were good enough to justify a Phase III clinical trial, set to begin in 1998. These trials will provide the higher dose to hundreds of volunteers.[21, 22]

The therapy's successes lend strong, albeit indirect support to the idea that leaky gut syndrome or dietary factors may trigger some cases of rheumatic disease. Oral tolerance therapy is not currently used in conventional clinical practice. Interested physicians and patients can contact Autoimmune Inc. of Lexington, Massachusetts, the makers of Colloral.

CHAPTER 11

VITAMINS AND MINERALS

LIKE THE GENERAL POPULATION, but to a greater degree, arthritis patients are deficient in key nutrients, vitamins, and minerals.[1,2] The documented shortages include nutrients known to be helpful in supporting normal immune function and minimizing inflammation. It is not always clear whether these deficiencies contribute to rheumatic diseases or result from the extra nutritional demands imposed by chronic inflammation. Regardless, it certainly makes sense to supplement your diet to ensure adequate intake of selected nutrients. This is especially true of the nutrients reviewed in this chapter.

We have listed the nutrients with the greatest therapeutic potential in alphabetical order, starting with vitamins. The most promising nutrients are vitamins C, D, and E, along with boron, selenium, and zinc, but you should look for multivitamin products that offer all of the nutrients described at or near the suggested doses. Supplement your multivitamin with individual nutrients as necessary.

VITAMIN A/BETA-CAROTENE

On average, people with rheumatoid arthritis have below-average blood levels of beta-carotene, the antioxidant plant pigment from which the body makes vitamin A. A new study from Johns Hopkins University indicates that low blood levels of beta-carotene (and vitamin E) may make people more vulnerable to rheumatic diseases. Researchers led by George Comstock, M.D., examined twenty thousand people in 1974. Compared with people who later acquired rheumatoid arthritis, beta-carotene levels in the blood of disease-free people were 29% higher. Arthritis and lupus patients had low levels of vitamin A and vitamin E, too, but only the differences in blood beta-carotene levels were significant.[3]

Does this apparent preventive effect extend to vitamin A intake? While vitamin A is critical to strong immune function, there is some evidence that high doses of vitamin A may aggravate damaging autoimmune activity. It seems wiser to consume supplemental beta-carotene, which the body uses to make only as much vitamin A as it needs. Meats, liver, eggs, dairy products, and fish liver oil are all high in vitamin A. In addition, diets high in meats and dairy foods appear to aggravate rheumatoid arthritis. If you eat these foods regularly and have rheumatoid arthritis, consider cutting your consumption and favoring foods rich in beta-carotene. These include leafy cooking greens (spinach, chard, kale, collards, etc.) and all red, orange, or yellow fruits and vegetables. Consider taking supplemental beta-carotene rather than supplemental vitamin A.

Note: High doses (20 mg/day) of beta-carotene may increase the risk of lung cancer moderately. It may be safer to obtain supplemental beta-carotene from "mixed antioxidant" formulas that contain additional carotenoids (lycopene, alpha-carotene, etc.) plus other antioxidants (e.g., vitamins E and C).

Vitamin A is measured in international units (IU) or retinol equivalents (REs). Beta-carotene is usually measured in milligrams. Adult men or women need 5–10 milligrams of beta-carotene. Adult men should take 5,000 IUs per day of vitamin A (1,000 REs). Adult women need 4,000 IUs per day of vitamin A (800 REs). Caution: Doses of vitamin A more than 10,000 IUs per day can cause birth defects. Pregnant women should get supplemental vitamin A from mixed carotenoid supplements.

B VITAMINS

Certain of the B-complex vitamins may offer some benefit to arthritis patients. In 1949, an uncontrolled study among 455 osteoarthrosis patients found that a daily dose of niacinamide (400–2,250 milligrams) significantly improved range of motion in various joints.[4] A placebo-controlled trial published in 1955 showed improved range of knee motion after six weeks of supplementation with niacinamide.[5] A well-controlled study, conducted forty years later by the National Insitutes of Health, found that a 3,000-milligram daily dose (500 milligrams six times a day) led to a 29% improvement in global arthritis symptoms among seventy-two osteoarthrosis patients.[6]

Deficiencies of vitamin B_5 are associated with cartilage degeneration and decline in direct relation to the severity of rheumatoid arthritis symptoms, but a 1963 study in Britain indicated that supplementation could provide only short-term relief of rheumatic symptoms.[7] A later, uncontrolled study of subjects taking pantothenic acid (25 milligrams each day) and a B-complex supplement showed significant but temporary improvement within one to two weeks.[8] Vitamin B_{12} may help normalize the activity of T cells, which are known to be key players in autoimmune attacks in rheumatic diseases.

To ensure adequate intake of all the B vitamins, take a multivitamin supplement containing the recommended daily allowances (RDAs), which should be indicated on the label. Seek medical guidance before taking higher doses of niacinamide or pantothenic acid. Note: People experimenting with therapeutic vegetarian diets need to take B_{12} supplements to ensure adequate intake.

VITAMIN C

In 1757, the British physician Joseph Lind conducted the first controlled clinical trial in history. Ignored and even suppressed for thirty years, his pioneering study proved that citrus fruits prevent scurvy—a serious disease characterized by degeneration of connective tissues, including cartilage. In the 1920s and 1930s, scientists finally identified ascorbic acid as the mysterious antiscurvy nutrient and designated it "vitamin C." What can vitamin C do for arthritic conditions?

A landmark study at Boston University suggests that vitamin C has significant preventive and therapeutic benefits. Over an eight-year period, researchers examined the effects of vitamins C and E in 640 older people, half of whom showed some signs of osteoarthrosis and half who did not. Those who consumed the highest levels of vitamin C (from food and/or supplements) were three times less likely to suffer osteoarthrosis or see a worsening of existing symptoms. They also had much less joint pain. Vitamin E and beta-carotene imparted far less benefit.[9]

Vitamin C is critical to the synthesis of new collagen in cartilage, and elderly people with cartilage disorders have been found to be deficient in vitamin C.[10] It was proved long ago that arthritis patients tend to have low levels of vitamin C in their blood and synovial fluid, perhaps because it is depleted by inflammations. People with an above-average intake of vitamin C have a lower risk of osteoarthrosis.[11]

Vitamin C also protects antiprotease enzymes, which help keep certain enzymes involved in inflammation from dissolving healthy cartilage (see the discussion of OPC, Chapter 13).[12] And the vitamin stimulates the formation of anti-inflammatory prostaglandins (PGE$_1$) that aid in the normal synthesis of collagen and other important components of cartilage.[13,14] Moreover, the body needs vitamin C to make corticosteroid hormones that help dampen runaway inflammations.[15] As this discussion makes clear, vitamin C is critical to cartilage health and helps protect against the ravages of chronic inflammation in all connective tissues.

It is important to eat lots of citrus fruits and vegetables and take 500 milligrams per day. Increase the dose as needed, up to 5,000 milligrams, until you feel a therapeutic effect. You may be able to take less vitamin C (250–2,500 milligrams) with equal therapeutic effect if you are also taking OPC (25–50 milligrams) every day (see Chapter 13).

VITAMIN D

The brittle bones associated with osteoporosis have long been recognized as a risk factor for osteoarthrosis. The best preventives are exercise, avoidance of excess dietary protein, and adequate intake of calcium and vitamin D. A new study suggests that supplemental vitamin D can help. Boston University researchers followed the progress of 556 elderly persons with osteoarthrosis, taking periodic radiographs, interviews, and blood tests over an eight-year period. They found that osteoarthrosis of the knee was three times more likely to get worse among the participants who averaged 200 units of vitamin D per day—the current U.S. RDA—compared with participants who averaged 386 units per day.[16] (They did not determine whether low vitamin D intake increases the risk of osteoarthrosis.) As a result, the researchers recommended that osteoarthrosis patients supplement their diets with 400 IUs of vitamin D per day.

The body makes vitamin D when it is exposed to sunlight, and it is available from certain foods, including meats and fortified milk. It seems wise for people with osteoarthrosis and anyone older than forty to take supplemental vitamin D. It is possible to overdose on vitamin D; do not exceed the amount recommended here. Men and women need 400 IUs per day. This dose equals the U.S. RDA for people under 50, and it is double the U.S. RDA for people over 50.

VITAMIN E

Vitamin E is a strong antioxidant protector of cell walls, with moderate but well-proved anti-inflammatory properties. The results of many animal studies and several clinical studies suggest that vitamin E can be of benefit to arthritis patients, who are often deficient in this antioxidant vitamin.[17] Clinical trials using moderate to high supplemental doses (400–1,200 milligrams per day) have shown significant improvement in pain and swelling.[18–21] In one study, vitamin E proved superior to the NSAID diclofenac and had fewer side effects. Vitamin E is a potent antioxidant and mild blood thinner with cardiovascular benefits. Doses over 400 IUs should be taken only with a doctor's guidance.[22] A safe dose is 400 IUs per day or up to 800 IUs per day under a doctor's supervision. Food sources include vegetable oils, nuts, seeds, and wheat germ.

BORON

This little-known trace mineral is lacking in many people's diets and is essential to the production of vitamin D. While its benefit to arthritis patients remains uncertain, boron has proved quite effective in relieving osteoarthrosis symptoms in one small clinical trial and in the published observations of an Australian rheumatology clinic.[23, 24] Boron has also been shown to limit loss of calcium and magnesium while enhancing the effects of estrogen in women—effects that tend to help prevent the osteoporosis that often accompanies osteoarthrosis in older women. Fruits and vegetables are the best food sources. A well-balanced diet may supply enough, but it will not hurt to supplement your diet with 3 milligrams per day.

COPPER

People with rheumatic diseases tend to have high levels of copper both in their blood and in synovial fluid full of oxygen radicals. Copper may enhance the effects of ceruloplasmin, which is a potent scavenger of the oxygen radicals that help cause damaging inflammation.

Copper is also a key element in copper-zinc–superoxide dismutase, an enzyme that protects against damage by superoxide free radicals. Copper may help control rheumatic inflammations, but this is far from clear to medical researchers. Accordingly, there is no reason to take high amounts of copper, which can interfere with zinc absorption. Copper bracelets are one of the oldest folk remedies for inflammatory types of arthritis. While sweat can cause copper to leach into the skin, there is no reliable evidence that such bracelets provide benefit (see Chapter 16).

Copper deficiency is exceedingly rare, but it will not hurt you to take supplemental copper as anti-inflammatory insurance. Take 2 milligrams per day and no more unless recommended by your naturopath or your physician—higher doses could interfere with the positive effects of selenium and zinc.

SELENIUM

Often found lacking in modern diets, this essential trace mineral is needed to make the key antioxidant enzyme called glutathione peroxidase. Osteoarthrosis patients seem to have significantly lower blood levels of glutathione peroxidase, which can be raised with supplemental selenium. Some studies suggest that supplemental selenium has significant anti-inflammatory and analgesic benefits in arthritis patients.[25]

Many arthritis patients in Europe use selenium–ACE, a selenium supplement with added vitamins A, C, and E. The clinical findings using this combination are mixed. A six-month clinical trial in England found that selenium–ACE provided no measurable benefit; but another clinical trial, in Australia, found benefit from taking a combination of selenium (140 micrograms) and vitamin E (100 milligrams).[26–28]

There are no especially reliable food sources of selenium. The U.S. RDA for adults is 70 micrograms (note micrograms, *not* milligrams), and it may be wise to supplement your diet with 50–200 micrograms of selenium (as selenium dioxide) per day as insurance. Do not exceed 200 micrograms per day without a doctor's guidance and avoid the riskier inorganic form called sodium selenite.

ZINC

The diets of arthritis patients are often deficient in zinc. This essential trace mineral may help by inhibiting the release of the inflammatory mediator histamine from immune cells. The results of one clinical study indicated that zinc decreased inflammation and stiffness in rheumatoid arthritis patients who failed to benefit from NSAIDs and other anti-inflammatory drugs. But other studies have not supported these positive findings, which may mean that zinc's usefulness is limited to certain drug-resistant or zinc-deficient patients.[29–31]

The U.S. RDA for adults is 12–15 milligrams, levels that may be obtained from a good multivitamin–mineral supplement. All available evidence suggests that it is safe to take as much as 30 milligrams per day. Caution: Zinc competes with copper for absorption, and for this reason it is important that supplemental zinc be accompanied by supplemental copper (see earlier discussion). Daily doses of zinc totaling 100 milligrams or more have been shown to be accompanied by unhealthful changes in blood cholesterol.[32]

CHAPTER 12

TRADITIONAL HERBS

DURING THE FIRST HALF OF THE nineteenth century, chemists discovered how to isolate and modify chemicals found in medicinal herbs and other natural materials. Today, one-quarter of all medicines still contain active ingredients based on chemicals found in plants. From a medical standpoint, herbs and synthetic medicines are both considered drugs, but there are often meaningful differences between them. Synthetic drugs typically contain concentrated amounts of one or a few chemicals, which increases the potential for toxic or unbalanced effects. This is why many drugs cause more adverse reactions than comparable herbs. A few herbs are about as fast-acting, potent, and toxic as their synthetic counterparts, but most of the herbal extracts that we will review in this chapter are safer and slower-acting than their synthetic counterparts. Most are not supported by as much scientific research as the approved arthritis drugs. This deficiency is balanced by their long histories of safe, effective use.

When the price of avoiding side effects is a more gradual, less dramatic benefit, it seems worth paying. This is especially true with chronic conditions such as arthritis, where patients may need to live with a drug and any side effects for a long time. Remember that synthetic drugs are not always fast-acting. The standard second-line arthritis drugs take weeks to months to produce relief, if they yield any at all.

Plant-derived nutraceuticals, such as curcumin and OPC, are covered separately (see Chapter 13) because these plant substances are not extracted from traditional arthritis herbs and contain a far narrower range of chemicals than the herbs. In contrast, most of the herbs discussed in this chapter have had long histories of effective use in relieving arthritis.

RANKING HERBS FOR ARTHRITIS

Any attempt to select the best herbs for arthritis is a judgment call. Accordingly, we have divided the herbs into two categories—primary therapeutic herbs and secondary herbs. In particular, the primary therapeutic herbs can complement physical and mental therapies and may match or exceed the benefits and safety of standard synthetic drugs. For those who want to know more, detailed scientific summaries of research on the primary herbs can be found in Appendix C.

There are many other herbs that hold significant promise for arthritis but lack substantial scientific or historical backup. Some of these herbs are listed in Appendix B, with an indication of their biological properties and place in traditional healing systems. It should be said that in any individual case, one or more of the herbs listed in Appendix B might prove more effective than the ones featured in this chapter. We chose the ones covered here for the reasons stated, in an attempt to help medical consumers sort through the hundreds of possibilities.

PRIMARY THERAPEUTIC HERBS

Many herbs can be said to provide benefit in rheumatic diseases, but certain ones offer the best history of traditional use or scientific proof of efficacy. Most of the top candidates come from India or China, in part because these nations boast the oldest and most highly developed systems of medical practice and botanical pharmacy in the world. The main pharmacological (drug) effects of each herb are listed under their headings (anti-inflammatory, cartilage protective, etc.). Whenever there is any doubt, the term is followed by a question mark.

BOSWELLIA SERRATA
(Indian frankincense)
ANTI-INFLAMMATORY • CARTILAGE PROTECTIVE

This ancient herb is one of the most exciting rediscoveries in botanical treatment of arthritis inflammation. The history of boswellia—a close cousin of the biblical frankincense plant—stretches back some four thousand years, to ancient Egypt. Based on current research, this ancient herb has a very bright future. The primary active ingredients are two boswellic acids.

Ayurveda and Arthritis

Ayurveda is a sophisticated medical tradition with roots as old as the dawn of Hindu culture more than three thousand years ago. Today there are more than one hundred Ayurvedic medical colleges in India and in excess of 300,000 practitioners trained in the tradition's herbal and dietary therapies. Even the World Health Organization recognizes Ayurveda ("the science of life span") as a repository of unique and valuable medicinal herbs.[1] Records of boswellia's properties date back to 700 B.C. when the paired pillars of Ayurvedic medicine were written. Both of these texts—the Sushruta Samhita and Charak Samhita—praise the *salai guggul* (resin) from *Boswellia serrata* as a superior antirheumatic medicine. All of the research relating to boswellia and inflammation employed modern extracts derived from the salai guggul described in these ancient texts.

Boswellia: Safety and Efficacy

Boswellia is a very safe botanical extract, as shown by its two thousand-year-long tradition, laboratory tests, and approval by U.S. and European authorities for use as a spice or seasoning.[2] Unlike NSAIDs, boswellia does not cause gastric ulcers and bleeding, changes in blood chemistry, or detectable adverse effects in any organs.[3-6] Indian researchers have examined the specific effects of boswellic acids in animals and people, with the excellent clinical results summarized in Appendix C. A safe dose of boswellia consists of 600 milligrams per day (200 milligrams three times a day), based on products containing about 65% boswellic acids.

GINGER
(*Zingiber officinale*)
ANTI-INFLAMATORY • ANALGESIC

How could this everyday spice, the stuff of soda pop and holiday cookies, be of any use to someone with serious arthritis pain? The question ought to be reversed. Ginger is an inexpensive, surprisingly effective reliever of inflammation-induced pain, with many other health benefits, no side effects, and a very long history as an antirheumatic medicinal food in China.[7] So why is it virtually unknown as an arthritis treatment in the West? There are three reasons. First, the research into ginger's unique, multifaceted anti-inflammatory properties is not well known to the public or doctors in the West. Second, dosage is key—take too little or take it inconsistently, and the results may disappoint. And, third, sad to say, familiarity breeds scientific disinterest.

Ginger, the Safe NSAID

As described in Chapter 3, inflammations start when immune cells kick off one or more of several cascade reactions that yield inflammatory mediators (leukotrienes and certain prostaglandins). Like boswellia, ginger inhibits, in part, the 5-lipoxygenase enzyme and its inflammatory cascade reaction. Ginger also partly blocks the COX enzymes, but unlike the synthetic NSAIDs, ginger does not fully block COX-1 and does not create gastric bleeding or stomach upset.[8] To the contrary, ginger has been found to lessen stomach acid and prevent ulcers from stomach irritants in rats.[9] In essence, ginger acts to maintain a healthy balance of inflammatory mediators—reducing excesses that lead to pain and tissue damage.[10, 11]

Ginger as Ace Antioxidant

In addition to blocking inflammatory cascade reactions, ginger diminishes runaway inflammation through its antioxidant activity. (Antioxidants are chemicals that neutralize free oxygen radicals.) Ginger contains antioxidants of extremely high potency (including the nutraceutical curcuminoids discussed in Chapter 13). In fact, whole ginger beats curcumin, vitamin E, and the food preservative BHA as a scavenger of damaging radicals called "peroxides." It is no wonder that a Japanese drug company recently patented an anti-inflammatory drug derived from the aromatic compounds in ginger (gingerols).[12] To gain full benefit, it is important to consume the whole root. Capsules of dried ginger will suffice, but it makes sense to use plenty of fresh ginger in cooking too.[13–15]

Effective Enzymes

Supplemental proteolytic (protein-digesting) enzymes, such as bromelain, may be very effective in relieving inflammation by dissolving immune complexes (see Chapter 13). If so, fresh ginger may be the cheapest food source, since it is extraordinarily rich in a potent proteolytic enzyme called zingibain.

Ginger: Safety and Dosage

Little needs to be said on the subject of safety. Ginger has been used as a food and tonic for thousands of years and is widely consumed in the United States for motion sickness and stomach upset. Arthritis researchers have observed no side effects in any of the many test subjects who have taken ginger for more than two years. The doses provided here are based on the results of their studies. Patients who took amounts more than 3 grams reported faster, fuller relief. Some took as much as 50 grams of fresh root (1.8 ounces) without any side effects. Taking more than one or two grams on an empty stomach could produce a brief, harmless burning sensation. Ginger is known to increase menstrual flow when taken in extremely large quantities and has been used this way to induce abortion. Accordingly, it is wise to avoid it in large amounts (more than 1–2 grams a day) during the first trimester of pregnancy. A standard dose of ginger is 500 milligrams to 7 grams of powdered root or up to 50 grams of fresh, lightly cooked root.

SHOSAIKOTO
(Bupleurum falcatum / Ch'ai-hu)
Anti-inflammatory • Immune Modulation

This Sino-Japanese herbal formula has made headlines as a promising anticancer drug, but it has other properties of great interest in rheumatic diseases. East Asian herbalists have long used shosaikoto—one of a group of similar herbal formulas known as *kampo* medicines—to treat inflammatory and autoimmune conditions as well as liver disorders. (Kampo medicines are the Japanese versions of ancient Chinese formulas first imported to Japan during the Han dynasty.)

Modern research bears out the wisdom of this practice, demonstrating that in animals shosaikoto balances the functioning of the immune system and enhances the anti-inflammatory effects of the body's own corticosteroids. Shosaikoto contains seven herbs, and the synergy among them is key to its effects. For rheumatic diseases, one important ingredient may be "Bupf" (*Bupleurum falcatum*), a plant also known as *Bupleurum chinense,* or Chinese thoroughwax. Licorice appears likely to be the other key ingredient in shosaikoto, with proven benefits all its own.[16]

Safety

Shosaikoto has an ancient history of medicinal use, and the many animal experiments and human trials (on cancer) conducted to date have turned up no significant safety concerns. In a large Japanese study involving 260 cancer patients, shosaikoto increased participants' survival rate over a five-year period.[17]

Shosaikoto: The Formula and Finding It

Given its unique properties, shosaikoto is an antirheumatic drug worth serious consideration. The formula or its constituents should be available from Chinese or Japanese apothecaries and herbal importers (see Appendix A). If you cannot find prepared shosaikoto, a trained, licensed acupuncturist with herbal expertise (see Appendix A) can prepare it by combining the major ingredients in the traditional ratios, as follows: *Bupleurum falcatum / ch'ai-hu* (29%), *Piniella ternata / ban xai* (21%), *Scutellaria baicalensis / huang qin* (12.5%), *Zisyphus vulgaris /* jujube (12.5%), *Panax ginseng* (12.5%), *Glycyrrhiza glabra /* licorice root (8%), and *Zingiber officinale /* ginger root (4%). If you cannot find the other ingredients, try taking Bupf and licorice under guidelines set forth in *Oriental Materia Medica: A Concise Guide* by Hong-Yen Hsu and associates (see "Chinese Herbal Medicine" in Appendix A, for publishing information). An appropriate dose of *Bupleurum* would be 6–7.5 grams per day (based on safe use in cancer trials).[18]

LEI-GONG-TENG
(*Tripterygium wilfordii* / Thundergod Vine)
IMMUNE-MODULATING • ANTI-INFLAMMATORY • ADRENAL-SUPPORTIVE

This intriguing herbal drug imparts fast, impressive benefits in rheumatic disorders, especially rheumatoid arthritis and systemic lupus erythematosus (SLE). Perhaps more than any other herb, it seems to improve many symptoms and blood measures at once. But taking Lei-gong-teng also requires caution, and no one should take it without expert guidance (see "Dosage Guidelines" here and Appendix C). Nonetheless, the Chinese tradition of safe, effective use against rheumatoid arthritis, SLE, and other rheumatic conditions is so long and the modern clinical evidence so promising that we would be remiss in overlooking it.

Despite its toxic potential, Lei-gong-teng still has a better safety record than most of the slow-acting anti-arthritic drugs described in Chapter 8. Because use of Lei-gong-teng requires close medical monitoring, it is preferable to choose a licensed acupuncturist and herbalist who is also trained as a medical doctor or who is willing to work closely with your physician. If it is misused, whole extract of Lei-gong-teng root possesses the potential to cause serious damage to the heart and kidneys. The far safer "glycoside fractions" used in most clinical trials for rheumatoid arthritis and lupus can lead to various adverse effects—skin rashes, disruptions in menstruation, and gastrointestinal upsets—which disappear spontaneously during the course of treatment.

We asked two experts for their opinions. Dr. Pei Pei Wishnow, Ph.D., is an MIT-trained biologist and expert in traditional Chinese medicine. Dr. Zheng Zheng Zhang, M.D., L.Ac., is a highly trained acupuncturist and herbalist with long clinical experience in China and Japan. Both women expressed the strong opinion that Lei-gong-teng should be taken in concert with complementary herbs in a balanced formula devised by a knowledgeable Chinese herbalist, taking into account the patient's own circumstances.

Potent Antirheumatic Herb

Oriental Materia Medica (see "Chinese Herbal Medicine" in Appendix A) summarizes traditional knowledge on Lei-gong-teng and lists more than sixty scientific studies. A detailed scientific review by leading European researchers analyzes the effects of the various commercial extracts.[19] The main U.S. medical database (Medline) describes several more studies that support Lei-gong-teng's reputation, with American recent studies detailing the ways in which it fights the immune system imbalances of rheumatoid arthritis, including inflammation. To quote the most recent review, "Studies in laboratory animals have indicated that extracts of *Tripterygium wilfordii* Hook f suppress both immune and inflammatory responses and also effectively treat a number of models of autoimmune disease . . . components of *Tripterygium wilfordii* Hook f suppress immune responses by inhibiting transcription of cytokine genes, including interleukin-2 and gamma interferon."[20] The same investigators found that Lei-gong-teng acts in part as a COX-2 inhibitor, like ginger and the new, synthetic COX-2 inhibiting drugs discussed in Chapter 3.[21]

There is no doubt that Lei-gong-teng often has dramatic positive effects on rheumatoid arthritis and SLE, especially when symptoms are most active. The herb possesses anti-inflammatory properties and selective immune-modulating/suppressing effects highly relevant to treating both conditions. [22, 23]

Much of the test tube, animal, and human clinical work on Lei-gong-teng has used crude water or alcohol extracts of the whole herb, but other studies have employed refined "glycoside" extracts containing almost none of the toxic, therapeutically irrelevant alkaloids. The term glycoside is referred to in quotes here because there is no evidence that the root actually contains glycosides. The two main commercial "glycoside" extracts—called T2 and GTW—each contain different mixtures of compounds, primarily di- and triterpenoids.

A state-licensed acupuncturist with training in Chinese herbalism can help you obtain the herb, which is available in liquid extracts and tablets. The GTW fraction is commercially available in the form of 10-milligram tablets—with the recommended dose for rheumatoid arthritis being 60–90 milligrams per day for a 132-pound (60 kilogram) adult. The GTW extract is produced by the Institute of Dermatology, the Chinese Academy of Medical Sciences, and the Taizhou Pharmaceutical Factory. The T2 extract is produced by the Taizhou Drug Factory, Jiangsu Province.

Oriental Materia Medica gives guidance on the dosage and schedule of administration, based on the form (liquid, tablets), the severity of the illness, the therapeutic response to Lei-gong-teng, and the patient's age, weight, and health status. Chinese researchers report that proper preparation of Lei-gong-teng requires removal of the two outer cortical layers of the root and aging for one year. According to *Oriental Materia Medica,* maximum effect should be felt after three months of use. Thereafter, a maintenance dose of one-third to one-half the initial dose should be taken for at least one year. This guide also gives specifications to enhance Lei-gong-teng's effects by combining it with other herbs.

In a minority of patients, "glycoside" extracts (T2 and GTW) can impair production of sperm, give rise to skin rashes or stomach upsets, and disturb menstrual cycles—temporary effects that tend to disappear during the course of treatment. (As of this writing, the T2 and GTW fractions were not commercially available—you may be able to obtain them through a Chinese herb suplier or acupuncturist.)

While appropriate preparations have shown benefit in kidney conditions, improper use of whole extract of Lei-gong-teng root may do serious damage to the heart and kidneys. Recorded fatalities from improper use of Lei-gong-teng are believed to be due to kidney failure.

Lei-gong-teng should be used with caution, under close medical supervision, especially in children, the elderly, pregnant women, and persons with diseases affecting major organs. Again, it is safer and probably more effective to use this herb as part of a formula, always under the guidance of an experienced, state-licensed acupuncturist/herbalist, preferably a Chinese-born-and-trained practitioner with a medical degree earned here or in China.

DEVIL'S CLAW ROOT
(Harpagophytum procumbens)
ANTI-INFLAMMATORY (?) • ANALGESIC • ANTIGOUT

Devil's claw root has a long folk history as a digestive aid and analgesic among southern Africa's indigenous peoples, but it was not traditionally used as an antirheumatic herb. It was first introduced to Europe in 1953 and is widely used there for digestion and arthritis. Devil's claw appears to be a safe herb, based on its use in Africa, animal studies, and clinical trials. Germany's Commission E (a Federal review committee that evaluated many herbal medicines) found no evidence of significant adverse effects. The evidence for efficacy, however, is mixed. One study showed that devil's claw lowers levels of uric acid in the blood and thus may offer real benefit in cases of gout.[24] The French government allows sale of the herb as a folk remedy for painful joints, and clinical trials in China and France suggest that devil's claw may be effective in relieving pain and inflammation in osteoarthrosis and rheumatoid arthritis (see Appendix C).

An appropriate dose of devil's claw root is 1,500 milligrams (500 milligrams three times a day). Harpagoside, the characteristic compound that identifies true devil's claw extract, is used to define the potency of standardized extracts. It is important to note that harpagoside has little or no anti-inflammatory effect by itself.[25] Choose whole root extracts, standardized for harpagoside content, to ensure that you are really getting devil's claw.

SECONDARY HERBS

The herbs reviewed here may be of great benefit to some people with arthritis. They did not make our primary herbs list for one of two reasons: either the evidence of efficacy was not as strong or they lacked a significant history of traditional use in arthritis.

WILLOW BARK
(*Salicis* cortex)
ANTI-INFLAMMATORY • ANALGESIC • ANTIFEVER

Many medicinal herbs for pain contain the salicylates from which aspirin is made. Judged on potency, willow bark may be the closest natural counterpart to aspirin. This does not mean that it is the best natural anti-inflammatory analgesic alternative to aspirin and other synthetic NSAIDs. Based on centuries of use and modern clinical trials, willow bark is weaker than aspirin but has far fewer side effects, including less gastric bleeding. Some people with mild to moderate osteoarthrosis pain might be able to use willow bark tea or alcohol extract to eliminate or limit reliance on aspirin, thereby minimizing the risk of dangerous side effects.

The German government recognizes willow bark extract as mildly effective for "feverish illnesses, rheumatic disorders, and headaches" and sets the minimum active dose at 60–100 milligrams of salicin.[26] Reputable manufacturers of liquid herbal extracts should be able to tell you how much of their willow bark product you need to take to reach this dose. If you wish to purchase willow bark to make tea, consider that among the various subspecies on the herbal market, the ones richest in salicylates are *Salix purpurea, Salix daphnoides,* and *Salix fragilis.*

Note: Other traditional herbs for pain that contain significant amounts of salicylates include meadowsweet flower (*Spiraeae* flos) and balm of Gilead (*Populus tachamahacca*). With any of these salicylate herbs, your best guarantee of potency is to choose a standardized extract (capsule, dropperful, etc.) that lists the milligrams of salicin per dosage unit. A standard dose of willow bark is 1–4 milliliters of alcohol extract, three times daily, or a standardized dose containing 30 milligrams of salicin three times daily.

FEVERFEW
(Tanacetum parthenium)
ANTI-INFLAMMATORY • ANALGESIC (?)

Fresh and dried leaves from the herb feverfew have a history of folk use for arthritis. Despite a lack of evidence that feverfew can relieve arthritis pain, many arthritis sufferers in the United Kingdom take the herb and claim benefit.[27] Use of feverfew for arthritis pain has a rational basis—animal studies show it possesses significant antirheumatic properties. In test tube studies on rabbit tissue, feverfew lessened inflammatory activity by blood platelets and immune cells and kept blood platelets from sticking to collagen.[28] These actions may explain feverfew's folk reputation for relieving moderate arthritis symptoms.

The only controlled clinical trial of feverfew for arthritis conducted to date had negative results. It studied a group of rheumatoid arthritis patients whose symptoms were unresponsiveness to conventional drugs, however, and the amounts of dried leaves used (70–86 milligrams) were fairly small.[29] In 1991, the Canadian health authorities proposed that standardized feverfew products containing a minimum of 0.2% parthenolide (the active constituent) be recognized as moderately effective in cutting down the frequency and symptoms of migraine headaches.

The effective dose, if any, is uncertain. Clinical trials have used up to 86 milligrams of dried, encapsulated leaves and liquid or dry extracts standardized to contain 0.2% to 0.4% parthenolide. (Evidence suggests that parthenolide is not the active analgesic ingredient in feverfew, but it serves as a marker of extract potency.) Given the herb's relative safety, larger doses should be safe if taken under medical guidance and supervision.

CELERY SEED
(*Apium graveolens:* fructus)
ANTI-INFLAMMATORY (?)

Celery seed and celery seed oil have recent but fairly strong histories of folk use in Europe as antirheumatic agents and have become popular antirheumatic products in Australia.[30] Celery seed is also listed as a traditional antirheumatic herb by the British Herbal Pharmacopoeia and Germany's Commission E, although both of these respected bodies declare a lack of clinical evidence. There is also evidence that water extracts of celery stalk have significant anti-inflammatory effects in animals.[31] Be aware that celery seed is contraindicated in kidney disorders and that celery stalk can cause allergic or light-sensitivity skin reactions in some people. The effective dose is unknown (use manufacturer's recommended dose).

YUCCA
(*Yucca brevifolia* or *aborescens* / Joshua Tree)
ANTI-INFLAMMATORY (?) • ANALGESIC (?)

This famous desert plant has gained a reputation for its value in arthritis based on the positive results of one rather poorly designed clinical trial published in 1975. We review yucca here despite serious doubts about the reliability of the research, largely because it has gained a following among some patients and experienced naturopathic physicians. Authors of the sole clinical trial of yucca divided 149 patients into two groups. One group received a yucca extract; the other received a placebo. The results look promising at first glance, with 61% reporting some relief from pain, swelling, and stiffness versus 22% reporting some relief with the placebo.

Unfortunately, the study suffered from several weaknesses. The participants continued taking unknown amounts of unidentified medications, the evaluations used to compile final results were based entirely on the patients' testimonies, and the periods of treatment varied enormously, from one week to fifteen months. In addition, the study recruited some patients with osteoarthrosis and others with rheumatoid arthritis.[32]

The researchers used an extract featuring yucca saponins. These soapy glucoside compounds form the bulk of the plant's solids. Natural saponins, like those in yucca or wild yam (*Dioscorea* spp.) can be used as building blocks to make synthetic cortisone. Orally ingested yucca saponins, however, may be destroyed by digestive fluids and are of doubtful value in fueling the body's production of anti-inflammatory corticosteroids. Instead, the study's authors suggested that yucca saponins might alleviate pain resulting from degeneration of cartilage by blocking absorption of bacterial toxins from the gut. This theory has some experimental support, derived from test tube studies of the effects of related compounds (lipopolysaccharides) on bovine calf cartilage.[33]

Oral yucca is a very weak hemolytic, or dissolver of red blood cells, but it is approved as a nontoxic food substance (root beer flavoring) in the United States and should be safe in moderate doses. Patients participating in the 1975 clinical trial took four tablets daily of a commercial yucca product. The study's authors did not identify which part of the plant the extracts came from or the saponin dosage of each tablet.

Michael Murray, N.D., a respected authority on the clinical use of herbal medicines, recommends taking one-quarter to one-half teaspoon of liquid extract, 200–500 milligrams of solid extract, or 2–4 grams of powdered leaf (in capsules or as a tea).

CHAPTER 13

NUTRACEUTICAL REMEDIES FROM NATURE

IN RECENT YEARS, SCIENTISTS HAVE REDOUBLED their efforts to find new therapeutic and protective agents in nature. The results have included nutritional, food-derived substances with pharmaceutical (drug) effects. This dual nature explains the origin of the term nutraceuticals that is used to describe them. It can be difficult to draw clear lines between nutraceuticals and herbs, but the distinction has real meaning. For example, curcumin and capsaicin are of benefit in treating rheumatic diseases, but neither one comes from a traditional "arthritis herb." Their source plants contain small amounts of therapeutic chemicals that have been concentrated in dietary supplements. Other nutraceuticals, such as sea cucumber, have histories of therapeutic use but do not fit neatly into any traditional category of remedy.

EPA
(FISH, FLAX, OR HEMP OIL)
ANTI-INFLAMMATORY

EPA (eicosapentaenoic acid) is a polyunsaturated fat that is essential to human health. It belongs to one of two main categories of essential

139

fatty acids, called omega-3 and omega-6 fatty acids. Certain fish fats are rich in EPA—an omega-3 essential fatty acid—and the body can also manufacture it from an omega-3 fatty acid called LNA (alpha-linolenic acid; see "Indirect Sources of EPA"). EPA is among the best-researched and most widely promoted of all nutraceutical arthritis remedies. The bulk of the evidence indicates that it can provide moderate benefits for many people with rheumatoid arthritis.

How does EPA help? Among other things, the body uses EPA to make prostaglandins that tend to dampen inflammation (see Chapters 3 and 6). The available evidence suggests that when arthritis patients increase the ratio of EPA or LNA in their diets—relative to meat, dairy, and standard vegetable fats—painful inflammations gradually decline in intensity. Medical researchers have thought that vegetarian-type arthritis diets relieve symptoms of rheumatoid arthritis because they automatically increase the ratio of polyunsaturated fats like EPA to saturated fats. One controlled study, however, found no relationship between the changes in ratios of various fats in tissues and the degree of relief experienced by people eating vegetarian-style diets.[1]

The supplemental sources of EPA—various types of fish and seed oils—range widely in cost ($12 to $120 per month) and usually take three months to produce benefits. You will want to know the pros and cons of each one, so we will take a closer look at the evidence. Be aware that every source of EPA takes three months or more to give noticeable therapeutic benefits.

EPA FROM FISH

The body fat in most cold-water ocean fish is rich in EPA, and for this reason these fats have been packaged in capsules and tested in rheumatoid arthritis patients a number of times. The results have been quite positive. A Harvard University team reviewed many of the arthritis studies that have tested the effects of EPA fish oil capsules. They concluded: "Use of fish oil improved the number of tender joints and duration of morning stiffness at three months as analyzed by both meta- and mega-analysis."[2]

Most studies have shown that rheumatoid arthritis patients see improvement in joint tenderness and pain after taking 3–7 grams of fish oil (in capsules) for three to twelve months.[3] Some studies have also shown that patients were able to limit or stop taking NSAIDs following this therapy.[4] Other controlled trials have shown that fish oils lead to improvement in both the symptoms of psoriatic arthritis and in the total area of skin affected.[5]

Even though all the studies conducted to date have used fish oil capsules, there are three reasons why it makes sense to get EPA by eating fresh, lightly cooked cold-water fish instead. First, EPA capsules are quite costly. Second, research shows that most EPA capsules contain oxidized fats that can contribute to inflammation and promote various chronic diseases.[6] Last, eating fish twice weekly appears to afford significant protection against rheumatoid arthritis—at least among women studied.[7] In rough order of EPA content, the best fish sources are sardines, mackerel, herring, salmon, bluefish, and tuna. You can also get EPA by taking cod-liver oil in capsule or liquid form, but it may become partly oxidized during processing.

Caution: EPA promotes thinning of the blood, which is one reason it is believed to help prevent heart attacks. At the doses used in arthritis trials, however, it will significantly decrease blood clotting and increase bleeding time of wounds, as do many NSAIDs. (Omega-3s do not promote gastric bleeding.) Be sure to consult with your doctor concerning this aspect of taking EPA.

INDIRECT SOURCES OF EPA: FLAX AND HEMP

Unrefined oils from flax and hemp seeds are rich in an essential omega-3 fatty acid called LNA (alpha-linolenic acid), which the body converts to EPA. This conversion is not 100% efficient, so these plant oils do not raise blood levels of EPA as much as encapsulated fish oils do, per gram of oil ingested. In addition, the results of one controlled clinical trial indicate that the addition of flax or hemp seed oil to a standard American diet may not raise blood levels of EPA or lessen inflammation.[8] The problem is that Americans' diets are very high in vegetable oils whose digestion uses up the same enzymes needed to convert LNA to EPA. Fortunately, there is a way around this metabolic bottleneck. Another study showed that when people taking flax or hemp oil also cut way back on their consumption of standard vegetable oils (corn, safflower, sunflower), their blood levels of EPA rose to the heights seen in successful clinical trials of fish oil therapy.[9]

Unrefined flax and hemp oils are sold in opaque bottles to protect their delicate fatty acids from destruction by light. (Keep them refrigerated at all times.) Either oil can be taken by the spoonful or used in salad dressings and other uncooked dishes. Hemp oil is much tastier than flax oil, which is available in capsules for those who do not like its flavor. Flax oil can be purchased in most health food stores.

Hemp oil is more difficult to find in stores but is easily obtained by mail order (see Appendix A). Hemp is also known as marijuana, but the nutritional hemp oil sold in the United States is completely legal, safe, and nonpsychoactive. Hemp oil also contains about 2% GLA (discussed later), a bonus if you choose it as an indirect source of EPA.

CANOLA AND EPA

The unrefined, opaque-packaged canola oil sold in some health food stores is quite high in LNA, and it is much cheaper than flax or hemp oil. Standard, refined brands of canola oil are processed for use in cooking and are not reliable sources of intact LNA molecules that the body can convert to EPA. Use unrefined canola oils only for dressings and other uncooked dishes. Use olive oil or regular, refined canola oil for higher-temperature cooking (sautéing, stir-fries, baking). An effective dose of EPA is 1.8 grams per day in capsule form or one tablespoon of cod-liver, flax, or hemp oil per day.

GLA

(BORAGE, BLACK CURRANT, OR EVENING PRIMROSE OIL)

ANTI-INFLAMMATORY

Borage, black currant, and evening primrose seeds are rich in an anti-inflammatory fat called GLA (gamma-linolenic acid). The clinical evidence in favor of GLA is less consistent than that favoring EPA, but several trials suggest that GLA-rich oils significantly alleviate joint tenderness and morning stiffness.[10–14] GLA, however, is relatively costly. To obtain the effective daily doses used in successful trials (1.4–2.8 grams), you would need to spend more than $100 per month—which is five to six times the cost of the experimentally effective dose of flaxseed oil.

The body uses GLA, like EPA, to produce certain anti-inflammatory prostaglandins. GLA also cuts down production of inflammatory messenger chemicals (cytokines) by immune cells and moderates their effects on immune T cells involved in controlling inflammation.[15] There is some doubt about the wisdom of long-term use of GLA, since it increases tissue levels of inflammatory fats (arachidonic acid) and lowers blood levels of EPA.[16] All three of these oils are available at health food stores in capsule form. Note: Researchers who have conducted random tests of GLA supplements have found that some brands contain none at all. The solution is to purchase reputable national brands (see "Dietary Supplements," Appendix A). An effective dose is 1.4–2.8 grams of borage, black currant, or evening primrose oil per day in liquid or capsule form.

CMO

(CETYL MYRISTOLEATE)

ANTI-INFLAMMATORY (?) • CARTILAGE PROTECTIVE (?)

In the early 1970s, a U.S. government research scientist named Harry W. Diehl made an intriguing discovery. Employed by the National

Institute of Arthritis, Metabolism, and Digestive Diseases, Diehl is best known for synthesizing the sugar compound used in Dr. Jonas Salk's oral polio vaccine. Harry Diehl was deeply moved by a neighbor's painful, ultimately fatal struggle with rheumatoid arthritis. This experience prompted him to begin conducting arthritis research on his own. His personal initiative may have produced a major development in the treatment of inflammatory arthritis and osteoarthrosis— a promising compound called cetyl myristoleate, or CMO.

Most animal research into rheumatic conditions employs Sprague laboratory rats, which are highly susceptible to rheumatic arthritis when they are injected with heat-killed mycobacterium (see Chapter 14)—a preparation called Freund's adjuvant. Diehl tried and failed to induce arthritis in mice using Freund's adjuvant and discovered that other researchers had encountered the same phenomenon. Intrigued, he decided to see if the mice were being protected by some physiological factor. Diehl analyzed the mice and discovered that they contain cetyl myristoleate (CMO), a previously unknown fatty acid. To date, only two other species—sperm whales and beavers—have been found to harbor CMO.

In 1977, Harry Diehl received a "use" patent covering administration of CMO to treat rheumatoid arthritis. To his disappointment, he could not interest any pharmaceutical companies in conducting research—in large part because it is extremely difficult to protect a product patent for a naturally occurring substance. Feeling that he had hit a brick wall, Diehl turned to other interests. Then, several years later, he himself began to experience osteoarthrosis in his knees, heels, and hands. After long-term therapy with NSAIDs and cortisone, he was no longer able to tolerate their toxic effects and decided to try CMO on himself—with dramatic success. As friends and family with arthritis became aware of his experience, many asked to try it, usually with excellent results. By 1991, the Diehl family had brought CMO to market as a dietary supplement.

Anecdotal accounts of CMO's alleged benefits abound, and at least one large, well-controlled clinical trial has been conducted, by the Mexican physician Humberto Siemandi, M.D., Ph.D., an experienced research administrator for hospitals in Mexico and Poland. Dr. Siemandi's clinical trial recruited 431 participants diagnosed with various rheumatic diseases—mostly rheumatoid arthritis or closely related conditions.[17] The multicenter study was conducted over thirty-two weeks under the auspices of the Joint European Hospital Studies Program; it was designed and supervised by a committee that included experienced rheumatologists and biostatisticians from Mexico's Federal Department of Health. Dr. Siemandi's study has not yet been accepted for publication by a peer-reviewed journal, but it appears to be of good scientific quality—randomized, double-blind, and placebo-controlled.

FIRST CONTROLLED
CLINICAL TRIAL OF CMO

Participants in Siemandi's trial were divided into three groups: 106 received only CMO, ninety-nine received a "CMO-plus" regimen (CMO, glucosamine hydrochloride, sea cucumber, and hydrolyzed cartilage), and 226 received a placebo. Participants were prohibited from taking caffeine or tobacco, which, according to anecdotal reports, interferes with CMO's alleged anti-inflammatory, analgesic effects. Compliance with each treatment regimen was closely monitored, and more than 85% of the participants (382) completed the trial. Treatment response was measured by blood and radiographic tests as well as physicians' and patients assessments. The results, from all perspectives, were remarkable; 87.3% of the CMO-plus group met the well-defined definition of positive response to treatment versus 63.3% of the CMO group and 14.5% of the placebo group. Laboratory measures (e.g., total neutrophils, Westergren ESR) also showed statistically significant improvement in the CMO and CMO-plus groups compared with patients who took the placebo. Results like these for a pharmaceutical drug would be big news—especially if it had no adverse effects.

As of this writing, it is still unclear how CMO works. It seems likely that CMO acts in a fashion similar to the essential fatty acids EPA and GLA, which suppress inflammation through their influence on the inflammatory cascade reactions mediated by prostaglandins. But EPA and GLA have not imparted anti-inflammatory effects as dramatic as those seen in this trial, even when taken over much longer periods of time. Cetyl myristoleate is also said to assist in lubricating joints, which would explain its alleged benefits in osteoarthrosis. Excitement seems warranted, but it should be tempered with healthy skepticism. More research must be performed to confirm Dr. Siemandi's results and illuminate the mechanisms by which CMO may alleviate the symptoms of rheumatic diseases and osteoarthrosis. At present, CMO is being produced from various vegetable and animal fats. Check the label and price carefully to find the product that is least costly.

Participants in Dr. Siemandi's clinical trial took about 525 milligrams of CMO per day (175 milligrams three times daily, with meals). Best results were experienced by the group who also took 600 milligrams each of glucosamine, sea cucumber, and bovine cartilage per day (200 milligrams of each three times daily, with meals)—a regimen that would be quite costly over the long term. The glucosamine hydrochloride and sea cucumber given to participants are not ideal sources of GAGs; it makes sense to replace these with glucosamine sulfate (1,200 milligrams per day).

The easiest way to control the dosage is to purchase CMO in a form that contains measured amounts, such as soft-gel capsules. If you use a liquid or powdered form, you will need to know, or find out from the manufacturer, how many milligrams of CMO are in a given measure of volume, such as a teaspoon.

EMU OIL
ANTI-INFLAMMATORY

Aborigines have long used an oily fat from emus, Australia's ostrich-like, flightless birds, as a balm for bruises, aching joints, and inflamed tissues. Some early European settlers emulated the natives' reliance on emu oil, but until fairly recently, it remained in the realm of obscure folk remedies. In the mid-1980s, Australian researchers began analyzing emu oil to quantify its effects and discover the active ingredients. At first, they thought the fatty acids in emu oil might be inhibiting production of inflammatory mediators (prostaglandins and leukotrienes). The fatty acid composition of emu oil is quite similar to chicken fat, however, which is not strongly anti-inflammatory, and comparative tests using oils with higher concentrations of anti-inflammatory fats were far less effective than emu oil.

Michael Whitehouse of the University of Adelaide and Peter Ghosh of Sydney's Royal North Shore Hospital decided to investigate emu oil further. They tested emu oil's yellow pigment against arthritic inflammations in lab animals, with great success. They theorize that the pigment comes from anti-inflammatory chemicals in the birds' bile and natural diet (bilirubins, carotenoids, flavonoids, flavonols, etc.). If this is true, it would raise doubts about the anti-inflammatory powers of emu oil from animals raised on commercial feed. Following this achievement, Drs. Whitehouse and Ghosh tested emu oil in a human clinical trial, the details of which we could not obtain. One emu oil vendor claims the study documented a complete cessation of pain in fourteen days and virtually ended inflammation in seventeen days. If so, you should see good results within a month of sustained application—or demand a refund.

U.S. PATENT IS
NOT PROOF OF EFFICACY

The experiments conducted by Drs. Whitehouse and Ghosh persuaded the U.S. Government to award them patent no. 5,431,924 in July of 1995. In it, emu oil is recognized as being "an anti-inflammatory topical pharmaceutical composition" and "a method for the treatment of musculoskeletal or dermatological conditions arising from inflammatory reactions of environmental or systemic origins." The awarding of the patent means that the researchers produced adequate evidence that emu oil is a unique anti-inflammatory substance. It does not constitute official endorsement of any medical claims made for emu oil.

Even proponents admit that emu oil only works when the site of inflammation is close to the surface of the body. To be effective at all against internal inflammations, emu oil must be mixed with a "carrier," such as alcohol or essential plant oils, which will transport it through the skin to inflamed tissues. Clever manufacturers have also been formulating emu oil with methyl salicylate—a carrier whose status as a U.S. FDA-approved nonprescription topical analgesic allows painkilling claims to be made on behalf of the product. Together with emu oil's lengthy folk tradition, the U.S. patent provides a reasonable basis for trying this unusual remedy. Emu oil is available in some health food stores and by mail order (see Appendix A). Rub over inflamed joints or tissues as needed.

BOVINE TRACHEAL CARTILAGE
CARTILAGE PROTECTIVE • ANTI-INFLAMMATORY

There is a very limited but promising body of clinical research that indicates bovine (cow) cartilage can alleviate symptoms and may minimize tissue damage in cases of osteoarthrosis (see Chapter 4), rheumatoid arthritis, psoriatic arthritis, and scleroderma. Most of these hopes are based on preliminary studies on cartilage therapy by the late surgeon John F. Prudden, M.D., who is more famous for discovering the promise of bovine cartilage as an anticancer nutraceutical drug. In the late 1950s, Dr. Prudden proved that cartilage extracts from various animals can accelerate wound healing. Later he showed that bovine cartilage has potent anti-inflammatory and immune-modulating properties. And unlike cytotoxic antirheumatic drugs such as methotrexate, the immune-modulating properties of bovine cartilage do not hinder immunity against infections or cancers.

In the early 1970s, Dr. Prudden and his colleagues at Columbia University performed groundbreaking clinical studies of the effects of cartilage on rheumatic and other inflammatory diseases. This research demonstrated that bovine tracheal cartilage has unsurpassed therapeutic effects in several types of rheumatic disease. Dr. Prudden had this to say at the time, concerning its effects:

> Our working assumption is that Catrix [his experimental bovine cartilage preparation] . . . is acting by coating cellular membranes, thereby preventing autoallergicity [as in rheumatic diseases] by interfering with pathogenic antigen–antibody combinations. . . . These data [tests of mice given Catrix and disease bacteria] indicate that this is a unique substance that in some way manages to inhibit acute and chronic allergic responses without affecting resistance to infection. These are remarkably useful characteristics indeed in comparison with all other anti-inflammatory agents and immunosuppressants.[18]

Bovine cartilage contains peptides (protein molecules) that curtail formation of new capillaries—an effect called antiangiogenesis. This property may be of benefit in limiting the damaging overgrowth of a granulation tissue called pannus, which often grows over and damages cartilage in rheumatic joints.[19-22] Only injected doses can be expected to offer this benefit, since the antiangiogenic peptides in oral doses of bovine cartilage are destroyed during the digestive process.

RHEUMATOID ARTHRITIS

In 1971, Dr. Prudden and chemist Leslie Balassa conducted a study on the effects of bovine cartilage (Catrix)—an experiment that led to remarkable results in patients with rheumatoid arthritis. Their first subject was a 57-year-old woman who had no detectable cartilage destruction but who had become progressively crippled by rheumatoid arthritis over a period of fourteen years. They began by injecting her with a small subcutaneous dose (75 milliliters) of Catrix, which initially exacerbated swelling. After three months with no further injections, she experienced dramatic improvement that lasted for three and a half months. As Dr. Prudden described it, "[Catrix] converted a housebound invalid who could not get off the toilet by herself into a woman who shops for herself . . . painted her own garage, and who jumps rope for exercise." She returned on her own for repeat injections whenever pain returned, about every three months.[23]

Dr. Prudden then tried Catrix injections in nine patients with severe, advanced rheumatoid arthritis marked by great pain, stiffness, and joint immobility. Despite the fact that laboratory measures of disease activity (erythrocyte sedimentation rate, etc.) did not suggest any remission of the disease, the Catrix injections produced significant therapeutic successes. Six of the nine patients experienced "good" results, and three enjoyed "excellent" results, meaning complete remission or very significant alleviation of pain, swelling, and joint tenderness.[24] Afterward, Dr. Prudden's attention was diverted to the use of cartilage in cancer. Incredibly, no arthritis researchers picked up the ball.

In an interview with Dr. Prudden concerning his brief but intriguing work on rheumatoid arthritis, he had this to say: "I have doubts that bovine cartilage alone can cure this very powerful disease, and our study was too small to prove anything. But the results were certainly encouraging enough to warrant further clinical work and justify medically supervised experimentation by individuals afflicted with rheumatic diseases."[25]

PSORIATIC ARTHRITIS

No rheumatic disease causes more psychological harm than psoriatic arthritis, with its unsightly skin patches adding insult to the pain of inflamed finger and spinal joints. The disease appears to be caused by a flawed immune reaction to a physical, chemical, or bacterial injury to the skin. As in rheumatoid arthritis, ankylosing spondylitis, and

Reiter's syndrome, many people with psoriatic arthritis have an unusual genetic marker on the surfaces of their cells—HLA-B27, in this case. It also occurs more frequently in people with psoriasis or a family history of psoriasis and is typically treated with toxic drugs, such as gold salts, sulfasalazine, or etretinate.

Dr. Prudden treated thirty-nine patients with severe symptoms, all of whom had tried the leading drugs (cortisone, methotrexate, etc.) for psoriatic arthritis. He administered amounts ranging from 70 to 1,000 milligrams by injection over periods ranging from six weeks to one year. The outcomes were most encouraging. Twenty-two subjects (56%) enjoyed excellent results, and fifteen (38%) had good results. Of those who experienced excellent results, nineteen saw a total remission of symptoms, including disappearance of lesions and excess skin cells, for an average of five months and up to one year in some cases. In some patients, lesions would disappear from some areas and appear in others, but all eventually vanished. Of the patients who had good results, many improved further when treated with topical Catrix cream.[26]

WHY ISN'T CARTILAGE PRESCRIBED?

Like glucosamine sulfate, bovine cartilage is sold as a dietary supplement, which is a serious disincentive for drug companies to spend the $230 million or so required to gain approval for it as a drug. Still, it is disappointing that rheumatologists have not seen fit to conduct further research and use a product that seems to work very well without any side effects. Catrix, which is made by "predigesting" and sterilizing cartilage from bovine tracheal rings, is now available in capsules and topical creams. Up to 9 grams of oral bovine cartilage can be taken per day, based on Dr. Prudden's results in treating osteoarthrosis. Before his death in the fall of 1998, Dr. Prudden was working to reintroduce an injectable Catrix product—a project that may yet reach completion in others's hands.

CAPSAICIN
(*CAPSICUM* SPP.) / CHILI PEPPER
TOPICALLY APPLIED ANALGESIC

Capsaicin, the hot chemical in chilies, is a slow-acting but effective topical (external) treatment for pain. Well over one hundred clinical studies have been reported on the various effects of capsaicin, most involving its ability to alleviate pain. For unknown reasons, it appears that capsaicin has more effect on the pain of osteoarthrosis than on rheumatoid arthritis pain. Capsaicin works by stimulating the nerves to release substance P, a neurotransmitter needed to send chronic pain signals. When capsaicin is applied to the painful area daily, substance P is depleted from local cells, and most patients feel much less pain.[27] Some feel quick relief, and others may have to apply capsaicin several times a day for one to two months before obtaining good results. It can be irritating to the skin, and you must be very careful to avoid getting residue on your hands and then in your eyes or mouth. Capsaicin creams (e.g., Zostrix) are available in most drug and health food stores. Rub capsaicin cream into affected areas as needed.

CURCUMIN TURMERIC
(*CURCUMA LONGA*) / *RAJANI*
ANTI-INFLAMMATORY • ANTIOXIDANT

Curcumin is the main active constituent in turmeric, an Indian herb with an ancient history of medicinal use against inflammation. Known to India's Ayurvedic physicians as *rajani*, turmeric is most familiar to Westerners as the bright yellow element in curry powder. This delicious spice is a close cousin to ginger and has been used for millennia to flavor, color, and preserve foods. Curcumin is the collective name for the antioxidant pigments in turmeric, called curcuminoids— a group of safe, natural NSAIDs (see Chapter 3). As enjoyable as Indian curries are, whole turmeric contains only about 5% curcumin, making its anti-inflammatory action rather weak. Fortunately, you can now purchase standardized dietary supplements of turmeric that contain 95% or more curcumin.

Curcumin is similar to aspirin and other NSAIDs in that it blocks formation of the pro-inflammatory mediators produced by the cyclooxygenase (COX) and 5-lipoxygenase enzyme cascade reactions. As we saw in Chapter 3, synthetic NSAIDs cause gastric bleeding and blood clotting because they block the COX-1 cascade that creates the beneficial prostaglandin called $PGI1_2$. Curcumin is much safer than standard NSAIDs, because it blocks another COX-produced prostaglandin—the pro-inflammatory mediator called thromboxane (TXA_2). In fact, a German company has been awarded a U.S. patent no. 5,401,777 that covers use of curcumin to prevent or treat diseases associated with excessive formation of inflammatory mediators.

Curcumin has the added benefit of acting as a very powerful scavenger of the oxygen radicals generated by arthritic inflammations. In fact, the substance far outstrips vitamin E and the potent fat preservative BHT (butylated hydrocoxytoluene) in protecting against destructive lipid peroxide radicals and rivals grape skin OPCs in that regard.[28–30] In addition, turmeric contains a protein (peptide) called turmerin, which is an even more powerful free radical scavenger than curcumin or the synthetic antioxidant BHA (butylated hydroxyanisole).[31] Like the Chinese herb Bupf (see Chapter 12), curcumin may also enhance the production of internal corticosteroids, or boost their anti-inflammatory power.[32, 33] Numerous animal studies have demonstrated curcumin's anti-inflammatory effects. These results led to the two positive clinical trials, including one testing curcumin against phenylbutazone, a potent synthetic NSAID.

CONTROLLED CLINICAL TRIALS OF CURCUMIN

In 1980, Indian scientists tested curcumin in forty-nine patients with rheumatoid arthritis. Half were given 1,200 milligrams of curcumin per day, and the rest received a standard dose of the potent synthetic NSAID phenylbutazone. At the end of six weeks, both groups experienced similar improvement in morning stiffness and physical endurance.[34]

Six years later, the anti-inflammatory potency of curcumin was tested in hospital patients who had either undergone surgery or suffered some kind of physical trauma. One-third received curcumin (1,200 milligrams per day), one-third were given a placebo, and one-third took phenylbutazone (300 milligrams per day) for three to five days. Curcumin was judged to be as effective as phenylbutazone.[35] A standard dose is 1,200 milligrams per day (600 milligrams taken twice a day). Look for turmeric supplements standardized to contain 90% or more curcumin.

OPCs

(GRAPE SKIN EXTRACT, PINE BARK EXTRACT, PYCNOGENOL)

ANTI-INFLAMMATORY • ANTIOXIDANT • COLLAGEN PROTECTIVE

In 1535, sailors on Jacques Cartier's expedition to Canada fell seriously ill with scurvy. This degenerative disease of connective tissues was caused by the typical seafarer's diet of the day—a nutritionally deficient menu consisting of dried meat and biscuits. The crew was saved by an Indian's advice to drink tea made from the bark of a certain pine tree. In the 1930s, when ascorbic acid was proved to be the elusive antiscurvy nutrient in certain fruits and vegetables, it was named vitamin C. To scientists contemplating Cartier's rescue, the slim vitamin C content of pine bark had always seemed insufficient to explain the rapid recovery of his scurvy-ridden crew.

In fact, vitamin C was not the miracle that saved Cartier and his company. For more than fifty years, European biochemists have been conducting research into Cartier's true savior—a family of antioxidant plant compounds called oligomeric proanthocyanidins (OPCs) or pycnogenols. Supplemental OPCs have been used in Europe since 1950 to treat weak blood capillaries, postsurgical edema (swelling), cirrhosis, varicose veins, and diabetic retinopathy.[36] The early research into OPCs as a treatment for capillary fragility hinted at their potential value in connective tissue disorders, but this limited focus understates their therapeutic promise and, until recently, has distracted scientists from looking into broader uses for OPCs.

Some researchers call OPCs "vitamin C_2," because they restore the antioxidant function of vitamin C molecules worn out by free radical scavenging activities. Vitamin C is critical to immune functions and the health of connective tissue, making it and OPC valuable to people suffering from arthritis, cardiovascular disease, and other conditions involving degradation of connective tissue (e.g., joints, artery walls). As yet, there are no clinical trials to support this theory, but the laboratory findings described here suggest that OPC should be considered a promising therapeutic agent for osteoarthrosis and inflammatory rheumatic diseases.

COLLAGEN CROSS-LINKAGE

OPCs promote healthy cartilage by normalizing "collagen cross-linkage," which is a key part of its structural integrity. Collagen consists of twin, ladderlike spirals of proteins connected by steplike cross-links. In osteoarthrosis and rheumatoid arthritis, the new collagen often contains too many cross-links, producing thick, stiff, dysfunctional cartilage that is prone to injury. Excess cross-linkage is caused by two processes related to inflammation, which occur in osteoarthrosis and especially in rheumatoid arthritis. The first is internal production of excess free radicals. Free oxygen radicals are the unstable, dangerous molecules our bodies cannot live without and must handle with protective gloves in the form of enzymes. The second factor in excess cross-linkage is release of excess amounts of the collagenase enzyme that destroys old collagen to make way for new. During the course of inflammations, the synovial cells in joints often release so much collagenase that it wreaks havoc in healthy collagen. OPCs help reduce excess cross-linkage by neutralizing free radicals, protecting collagen from excess collagenase, and helping vitamin C support synthesis of healthy new collagen.[37–42]

ANTIOXIDANT/ ANTI-INFLAMMATORY ACTIONS

As we saw in Chapter 6, much of the cartilage damage that takes place in rheumatic diseases is created by superoxide free radicals, which are produced by inflammatory immune reactions. When it comes to scavenging oxygen radicals, OPCs are eighteen times more effective than vitamin C and fifty times more potent than vitamin E.[43, 44] In addition, OPCs refresh the antioxidant capacity of vitamin C molecules exhausted by free radical scavenging activities. In one experiment, OPCs boosted vitamin C activity by an amazing 1,000%.[45]

Work by European researchers strongly suggests that OPCs safely inhibit a broader range of inflammatory mediators than synthetic NSAIDs, without the attendant side effects. Like ginger, they are believed to block lipoxygenase and COX-2, but they may also inhibit the actions of key inflammatory mediators, including histamine, prostaglandins, kinins, and more.[46] The anti-inflammatory properties of OPCs have been proved in laboratory studies on test animals and in human clinical trials involving sports injuries and postsurgical recovery. OPCs have not been clinically tested against arthritic inflammations, but given their mode of anti-inflammatory action and affinity for collagen, they may be very useful in minimizing rheumatic inflammation and its resulting damage to connective tissues.[47–50]

FORM AND DOSAGE

At present, pine bark extracts rich in OPCs dominate the U.S. market. But grape skin extract contains equivalent amounts, including a unique antioxidant (B2-3'-o-gallate) that makes it a more desirable source. In addition, most of the research has been done on grape skin extract, and it is less expensive. OPCs are reported to generate better antioxidant effects in body tissues when they are packaged in a patented chemical envelope called a Phytosome. The envelope in OPC Phytosomes is made of phosphatidylcholine (lecithin), a harmless nutritional factor.[51] OPC Phytosomes are believed to be as effective as straight OPC extract, at half the dosage level. This enhanced efficiency must be weighed against the cost differential per milligram of OPCs. The standard dose is 200 milligrams per day for two weeks, followed by 25–50 milligrams per day. Alternatively, try OPC Phytosomes at half these dosages. Red wine and ripe fruits can contain significant quantities of OPCs.

DIETARY ENZYMES

ANTI-INFLAMMATORY • CLEAR IMMUNE COMPLEXES (?)

Enzyme therapy for rheumatoid arthritis is quite controversial, but it has been put to the test in several studies with good results. How could digestive enzymes help alleviate the inflammatory symptoms of rheumatic arthritis? Rheumatoid arthritis is linked to high levels of immune complexes in synovial fluid (see Chapter 6). Normally, immune complexes circulate in the blood, synovial fluid, or lymphatic fluid until they are consumed by immune cells called macrophages. With rheumatic diseases, however, immune complexes accumulate in connective tissues (blood capillaries, joints, skin, etc.) and attract immune system proteins called "complement." Complement proteins attach to antigens and attract immune cells that engender chemical attacks and consequent tissue damage. To make matters worse, a kind of scar tissue called fibrin covers the damaged tissues. Fibrin shields the remaining immune complexes as they continue stimulating autoimmune attacks.

Supplemental enzymes—especially the protein-digesting varieties—are believed to do four things that lessen inflammation, pain, and tissue damage: dissolve immune complexes, dissolve the fibrin envelopes around immune complexes, activate special immune cells that digest immune complexes, and disrupt inflammatory cascade reactions.[52-54]

DOUBTS ABOUT ENZYME THERAPY

Supplemental enzymes are not proved to consistently initiate any of the biological effects listed. As a result, most rheumatologists question the assumptions underlying enzyme therapy for rheumatoid arthritis. Writing in a 1985 journal article, one German researcher spoke for the doubters when he wrote that "enzyme mixtures, apart from the problems of absorption, only influence circulating immune complexes, and moreover, in many diseases neither the aetiology [cause] nor [the] pathogenesis is connected with the immune complexes, [so] this therapy concept can be regarded neither as [affecting] causal [factors] nor as scientifically guaranteed."[55]

IN DEFENSE OF ENZYME THERAPY

There are several flaws in the preceding critique.

- One-quarter of supplemental enzymes do survive digestion and make it into the bloodstream.
- If enzymes cannot get at immune complexes lodged in connective tissues—and this may not be true, judging by the results of the clinical trials—they can at least diminish the number of circulating immune complexes that would otherwise end up in connective tissues.
- At least in rheumatoid arthritis, fluctuations in the severity of symptoms follow fluctuations in the levels of immune complexes measured in joints.
- Last, there have been several clinical trials in Germany testing enzyme formulas against rheumatic diseases. The results, which

were published in peer-reviewed medical journals, were largely positive. Most American doctors are unaware of these studies, which are not available in U.S. medical databases. These studies were conducted after the scientific critique quoted above was published.

CLINICAL TRIALS: WOBEMUGO ENZYME FORMULA

Between 1985 and 1990, several digestive enzyme preparations called WobeMugo were tested in German clinical trials comprising almost 1,800 patients. These formulas were originally developed for use in cancer treatment and are weaker than formulas now available, but they still proved quite effective. One of these trials was double-blind and placebo-controlled, while two were controlled tests comparing enzymes to standard gold therapy. Most were uncontrolled, leaving significant doubts about the results. But overall the results seemed positive.

- Significant improvement was seen in the WobeMugo group, compared with placebo, in a double-blind, controlled, multicenter study of 424 patients with nonarticular rheumatic diseases.[56]
- Of 168 patients with nonarticular rheumatic diseases, 77.6% had good to very good results after six weeks on WobeMugo.[57]
- Thirty patients with rheumatoid arthritis-like symptoms were judged to have experienced distinct improvement after receiving WobeMugo for six weeks.[58]
- In a multicenter study of 1,004 patients, 67% enjoyed good to excellent results.[59]
- Forty-two patients with chronic rheumatoid arthritis were given WobeMugo for six weeks. Blood levels of rheumatoid factor and immune complexes were monitored. At the end, 62% showed significant improvement. Measured levels of immune

complexes in the blood correlated well to symptoms—the fewer the immune complexes, the greater the relief.[60]

- In two separate studies, WobeMugo was tested against injected gold and oral gold in 102 patients with diagnosed rheumatoid arthritis. Both groups showed comparable improvement in clinical measurements (grip strength, etc.), but the enzyme group had fewer side effects. The results were muddied by use of NSAIDs and SAARDs by some patients.[61, 62]

- Nine of ten patients showed clear improvement in symptoms after six weeks of enzyme therapy, with none reporting side effects.[63]

The German clinical trials employed WobeMugo formulas containing enzymes and rutin (a bioflavonoid antioxidant), in approximately these doses: 100 milligrams of pancreatin, 60 milligrams of papain, 45 milligrams of bromelain, 25 milligrams of trypsin, 10 milligrams of lipase, 10 milligrams of amylase, 1 milligram of chymotrypsin, and 50 milligrams of rutin.

WobeMugo is not available in the United States, but a slightly different formulation called Wobenzym N is marketed here by the same German manufacturer (see Appendix A). The only apparent distinction between WobeMugo and Wobenzym N is that the latter does not contain amylase or lipase (starch- and fat-digesting enzymes, respectively).

To ensure that you are getting your money's worth from any enzyme product, consult a practitioner who is fully conversant with enzymes and the different ways in which their digestive potencies can be measured. Because the effects of enzymes depend upon dosage, it makes sense to take more proteolytic enzymes than are found in WobeMugo. For example, pancreatin can be safely taken in doses of 10X/325 milligrams or more.

Note: As with NSAIDs or other anti-inflammatory drugs, the effects of enzymes are temporary. Enzymes must be taken continuously to maintain low levels of immune complexes, and they should be taken between meals for maximum effect.[64] Therapeutic doses of papain and bromelain can cause nausea, diarrhea, or allergic reactions in some persons—effects that may be ameliorated by taking enzymes with meals. There is no evidence that enteric-coated enzyme supplements perform any better than uncoated supplements.

ENZYME THERAPY WITH BROMELAIN

Bromelain, a mixture of proteolytic enzymes from pineapple stems, possesses proven anti-inflammatory properties that may impart real benefit.[65, 66] An uncontrolled clinical trial conducted in the mid-1960s tested the effects of bromelain in twenty-nine arthritic patients, twenty-five of whom were suffering from advanced rheumatoid arthritis and were being treated with corticosteroids. (The remainder had osteoarthrosis or gout.) After their steroid doses were gradually reduced, the participants were put on enteric-coated bromelain supplements and observed for up to thirteen months. Based on joint swelling and mobility, 28% had excellent results, 45% had good results, and 14% had fair results.[67] The bromelain therapy had no side effects and allowed most participants to decrease their maintenance dose of steroids.[68] An appropriate dose of bromelain is 20–40 milligrams taken three times daily, based on positive clinical results.

SEA CUCUMBER
(PSEUDOCHOLOCHIRUS AXIOLUGUS)
CARTILAGE PROTECTIVE (?)

Chinese physicians have been prescribing sea cucumber soup for joint and connective tissue pain for some five thousand years. This marine animal resembles a large cucumber, with a tough outer skin covering a flexible, shell-like crust. Dried, powdered, encapsulated sea cucumber has become a fairly popular dietary supplement for the inflammatory pain of rheumatoid arthritis and osteoarthrosis, especially in

Australia, where much of it is harvested. So far, no compounds with proven anti-inflammatory properties have been identified in the animal. It appears likely that some of its benefits derive from the animal's high content of GAGs—the building blocks of cartilage reviewed at length in Chapter 4.

There is some unpublished clinical research of uncertain quality that supports the Chinese tradition. A double-blind, placebo-controlled trial of sea cucumber was conducted by the Rheumatology Department of the University of Queensland, Australia, in 1988. Over a six-month period, eighteen patients with rheumatoid arthritis took 500 milligrams of sea cucumber twice a day, while sixteen controls took placebo capsules. The authors detected no toxicity or adverse effects, and they judged that sea cucumber had caused "less deterioration" in the experimental group compared with the placebo group.[69]

All of the available research has been conducted on *P. axiolugus*, the species used in traditional Chinese medicine and cuisine. Given its safe use as a food for thousands of years, there is no reason to believe that powdered, encapsulated sea cucumber presents any health threat. No one yet knows exactly how sea cucumber works, but its high GAG content and the strong Chinese tradition of efficacy suggest that it may be worth trying for a few weeks. A standard dose of sea cucumber is 500 milligrams twice a day.

NEW ZEALAND GREEN-LIPPED MUSSEL
(*PERNA CANALICULUS*)
ANALGESIC (?) • CARTILAGE PROTECTIVE (?)

Judging by the results of two clinical trials of uncertain quality, supplements containing this marine animal may alleviate the pain and improve the mobility of people with osteoarthrosis. The evidence is thin. To quote from the respected reference book, *The Honest Herbal*, by the noted scientific expert on natural drugs, Varro Tyler, Ph.D., scientific studies "have not produced any substantial evidence of the effectiveness of mussel extract for arthritis." Like sea cucumber, green-lipped mussel is rich in GAGs, the amino sugars that the body uses to build cartilage (see Chapter 4). But glucosamine sulfate is a cheaper source of GAGs and has much stronger clinical, laboratory, and safety records.

TWO CLINICAL TRIALS
OF MUSSEL EXTRACT

In a double-blind, placebo-controlled study, seventeen of thirty-three patients who were diagnosed with severe osteoarthrosis and who were resistant to pain relief by NSAIDs received commercial extracts of green-lipped mussel. Sixteen patients were given a placebo, and both groups continued to take NSAIDs. At the end of three months, all were evaluated using standard clinical measures. Half of the group receiving mussel extract had improved compared with 14% of the controls. After three months, all participants began taking mussel, and 29% of the controls experienced improvement. Side effects included minor nausea, flatulence, water retention, and temporary increased stiffness. The same researchers tested the effects of mussel extract in thirty-one osteoarthrosis patients for periods ranging from six months to four and a half years. Just over one-third were reported to experience some benefit.[70, 71] A typical dose of mussel is 1,050 milligrams per day.

CHAPTER 14

ANTIBIOTIC THERAPY

AS EARLY AS THE 1860S, DOCTORS BEGAN TO suspect that microbes (bacteria) and viruses cause the various rheumatic diseases. The hypothesis gained momentum through the 1930s, but subsequent difficulty in identifying the microbes responsible led to a gradual loss of scientific interest. By the close of World War II, the microbe hypothesis of rheumatic disease had been virtually abandoned.[1] Today, the tide has begun to turn. It is now established that infectious microbes cause certain forms of arthritis, and there is strong circumstantial evidence that microbes play a role in many cases of rheumatic disease.[2] In this chapter, we will explore the relationship between microbes and rheumatic diseases and the evidence that antibiotics may be a rational choice in select cases—despite known drawbacks.

BACTERIAL ARTHRITIS

Infections that become focused on joints can damage them directly and will elicit inflammatory attacks by immune cells, causing further damage. These localized infections are called "bacterial arthritis."

While they do not usually feature the autoimmunity that defines most rheumatic diseases, they can sometimes engender it. Examples of bacterial arthritis include Lyme disease, rheumatic fever, fungal arthritis, gonococcal arthritis, and tuberculous arthritis. The conventional treatment is a course of antibiotics. The role that microbes play in rheumatic diseases is less clear. If microbes are involved in the onset of some cases, they may be only one of several causes or cofactors. This fascinating detective story features a real medical hero and a finale that remains unwritten.

CLUES FROM THE HEART AND GUT

The theory that microbes cause many cases of rheumatic diseases has been bolstered by the startling discovery that microbes give rise to duodenal ulcers and may bring on cardiovascular disease. Together with research into the causes of arthritis and positive results of clinical trials testing antibiotic therapy, these discoveries have given the microbial theory of rheumatic diseases new life.

BACTERIA CAUSE ULCERS

For many decades, doctors blamed duodenal (intestinal) ulcers on stress, irritating foods, and excess acid. As a result, they prescribed counseling, bland diets, and drugs to minimize acid and coat the intestines. Then, in 1982, medical researchers J. Robin Warren and Barry Marshall discovered a microbe hiding between the lining and mucous membrane of ulcerous stomachs. They suspected that the bacteria, *Helicobacter pylori,* might be the root cause of duodenal ulcers. Dr. Marshall bravely tested the theory by ingesting a large dose of *H. pylori* and promptly developed a case of duodenal ulcers felt 'round the medical world. Subsequent research proved nine of ten duodenal ulcers are infectious in origin and can be successfully treated with a long, strong course of antibiotics.

BACTERIA MAY
CAUSE HEART DISEASE

Genetics, fatty diets, and smoking have long been identified as the chief causes of atherosclerosis—the fatty buildup that causes most heart attacks and strokes. But Dr. Joseph Muhlestein and his colleagues at the University of Utah were aware of several clues suggesting a bacterial factor in the onset of atherosclerosis. In June of 1996, the *Journal of the American College of Cardiology* published the results of Dr. Muhlestein's research—a study that sent tremors through the medical community.

The Utah team had examined the arteries of ninety patients with atherosclerosis and found that some 80% harbored a special strain of *Chlamydia* bacteria. In contrast, they found *Chlamydia* bacteria in the blood vessels of only 4% of the twenty-four participants with healthy cardiovascular systems. Dr. Muhlestein's group suspected that the bacteria might be only an opportunistic feeder on fatty, diseased tissues, but when they examined the vessels of patients with heart transplants—people who had a condition similar to but distinct from atherosclerosis—they found no *Chlamydia* organisms.

It remains unproved whether the bacteria produce atherosclerosis by themselves or simply accelerate a process initiated by genetic and lifestyle factors. In light of the sorry history of misguided ulcer treatment, researchers are scrambling to perform follow-up studies. Given the disappointing history of rheumatology, researchers are examining the old microbial theory of arthritis with renewed vigor.

HOW MICROBES MIGHT
CAUSE RHEUMATIC DISEASES

There are several ways in which microbes are believed to be capable of causing the autoimmune responses that define rheumatic diseases: molecular mimicry, hypersensitivity, and antibody deficiency.

MOLECULAR MIMICRY

Microbes sometimes use a protective camouflage called molecular mimicry. When accosted by an immune cell, they display a portion of themselves that resembles one of the host body's tissues. This act of deception can lead to a "cross-reaction," in which antibodies or immune cells begin to attack the mimicked body tissues (see "Leaky Gut Syndrome," Chapter 6). Cross-reactions resulting from molecular mimicry are strongly suspected to cause multiple sclerosis, rheumatic fever, diabetes mellitus, and some of the major rheumatic diseases.

HYPERSENSITIVITY

Some researchers believe that genetic flaws in the immune system allow microbial antigens to build up in body tissues. After years of irritation, the affected tissues may experience a hypersensitivity to the antigens that stimulates a chronic inflammatory immune response.[3, 4] Rats carrying the same genetic marker that is found on the cells of humans with ankylosing spondylitis (HLA-B27) show signs of the disease—but not when they are raised in a germ-free environment.[5]

Human immune cells with this genetic marker are hypersensitive to the elusive microbes known as "mycoplasmas," which have long been suspected of triggering rheumatic diseases.[6] This finding has yet to be tested on immune cells bearing the faulty HLA markers found in most people with rheumatoid arthritis, Reiter's syndrome, and juvenile arthritis (see Chapter 6). Ironically, the immune system's attempts to eliminate microbial antigens may trigger rheumatoid arthritis. The body's immune response leads certain microbes to hide in or on cells and structures in connective tissues.[7, 8]

ANTIBODY DEFICIENCY

In most infections, the role of antibodies is only to lock onto microbes, marking them for destruction by immune system cells.

When it comes to mycoplasma-type microbes, however, antibodies are responsible for disabling the invaders without help from immune cells.[9] Some people suffer a deficiency of antibodies, and they are known to be more susceptible to mycoplasma infections and rheumatoid arthritis.[10–12]

People with antibody deficiency have very few of them in their intestinal walls, which are key points of entry for mycoplasmas and other microbes. As one leading research team put it, "The role of antibodies is to control the growth of mycoplasmas on mucosal surfaces; neutrophils [immune cells that "eat" microbes] play no part in defense and may even aid dissemination of the infection."[13, 14] This immune deficiency can be treated with supplemental antibodies, and clinical trials have proved the therapy to be quite effective in alleviating symptoms in patients with severe rheumatoid arthritis.[15] Some researchers familiar with mycoplasmas and rheumatoid arthritis recommend trying a combination of antibody therapy and antibiotic therapy.[16]

EARLY EVIDENCE FOR MICROBE THEORY

As we will see later in this chapter, the strong responses of many patients to antibiotic therapy bolster the microbial theory of rheumatoid arthritis, but do not prove it. The search for further evidence begins with mysterious microbes suspected of triggering many cases of rheumatic disease.

MYCOPLASMAS
AND L-FORM BACTERIA

Near the end of the nineteenth century, an epidemic swept through Europe's cattle herds, leaving thousands of animals with pneumonia and inflammatory arthritis. When scientists put the guilty *Streptobacillus* germs under the microscope, they found that they were surrounded by smaller organisms that looked like jellyfish. These were the elusive "L-forms" that streptococci, brucellae, and certain other bacteria adopt under attack. The bacteria shed their cell walls, and their essential parts persist in the form of a gel (plasma), to give the organism a better chance of hiding from the host animal's defenses.

MYCOPLASMAS—FOUND AND LOST

In 1898, French scientists at the Pasteur Institute discovered a whole family of unique, elusive microorganisms that exist only in the L-form, with no cell walls. Like bacteria, blue-green algae, and other "prokaryotes," these primitive microorganisms lack a distinct nucleus. (All animals are eukaryotes, whose genetic material is organized within a distinct nucleus.) These chameleon-like microbes, called mycoplasmas, are neither bacteria nor viruses, and are very good at making themselves practically invisible. Even if a mycoplasma or L-form bacteria caused a case of rheumatic disease, the organism's evasion skills would frustrate attempts to prove it. Through the 1920s, researchers failed to pin rheumatoid arthritis on any known bacteria, although they had long suspected that mycoplasmas were implicated. Scientists were stymied by the extreme difficulty of isolating the elusive microbes from human tissues using the technology of the day. Then the legendary Dr. Albert Sabin, who later developed the oral polio vaccine, found that he could induce arthritis in mice by injecting them with mycoplasmas.[17]

DR. TOM BROWN'S BREAKTHROUGH

Inspired by Dr. Sabin's work, Dr. Thomas McPherson Brown set out to see whether mycoplasmas were the cause of rheumatoid arthritis. Dr. Brown's interest was piqued in part because he knew that gold salts and hydroxychloroquine—the leading rheumatoid arthritis drugs of the day—were exceptionally toxic to mycoplasmas. In 1939, following hundreds of painstaking attempts, Dr. Brown and a colleague at New York's Rockefeller Institute managed to isolate mycoplasmas from the synovial fluid and tissues of a woman with rheumatoid arthritis.[18]

At the time, most physicians were very receptive to the idea that microbes could be a major cause of rheumatoid arthritis, and the team's feat was hailed as a breakthrough. When other researchers failed to repeat these results after a handful of attempts, however, rheumatology researchers began to lose interest in microbes. Dr. Brown and a few colleagues had already had great success in relieving rheumatic symptoms with antibiotics and continued to refine and document the therapy in the course of clinical practice.[19] Dr. Brown endured decades of professional isolation, even though his antibiotic therapy worked well for legions of patients who found their way to his Arthritis Institute at the National Hospital in Washington, D.C.

For ethical reasons, Dr. Brown refused to conduct placebo-controlled trials that would leave half of the participants untreated for long periods, yet there is credible, peer-reviewed evidence from retrospective studies to support the efficacy of his work with antibiotics.[20] And none of Dr. Brown's more than ten thousand patients ever sued him for malpractice, despite his reliance on a therapy opposed by an aggressively antagonistic medical establishment. On the contrary, hundreds of his patients volunteered testimonials to the superiority of antibiotic therapy—especially compared with previous unsuccessful treatment with conventional drugs (see The Road Back Foundation under "Antibiotic Therapy," Appendix A).

THE CHANGING FORTUNES OF MICROBE THEORY

In 1950, two American doctors undertook a risky experiment in which healthy human subjects were injected with synovial fluid from rheumatoid arthritis patients. Fortunately for the subjects, this ethically questionable test failed to induce rheumatoid arthritis—an outcome that weakened the microbe theory of rheumatic diseases.[21] The next high-profile test came in 1971, when a year-long clinical trial at Boston University found no improvement in rheumatoid arthritis patients taking tetracycline antibiotic.[22] The group studied was very small, and most observers considered the trial inconclusive. But the National Institutes of Health (NIH) was under congressional pressure to issue a report on progress in arthritis therapy and made a hasty, generally negative assessment of microbe theory and antibiotic therapy. Unfortunately, this report by the government's main research body discouraged many scientists from conducting further research.

Fortunately, the NIH report did not discourage all researchers. Interest in microbe theory persisted among some scientists, and a trickle of intriguing findings continued to keep it alive.

- Researchers at the NIH injected synovial fluid from a rheumatoid arthritis patient into the joints of three chimpanzees. This test produced rheumatoid arthritis symptoms in the apes, and synovial fluids from the human patient and the chimps both contained antibodies to mycoplasmas.[23]
- Latin American researchers reported good results from a small, uncontrolled trial of tetracycline in rheumatoid arthritis.[24]
- American doctors published the first of several studies documenting the presence of mycobacteria—germs similar to mycoplasmas—in tissues of patients suffering from the deadly rheumatic disease scleroderma.[25]
- New studies showed that microbes commonly cause rheumatoid arthritis and other rheumatic diseases in chimpanzees, rats, swine, poultry, and various domestic animals.[26–28] The guilty parties were mycoplasmas and *Chlamydia*—a parasitic bacteria that produces a rheumatic disease (Reiter's syndrome) in the connective tissues of genetically susceptible people.
- Throughout the 1980s and 1990s, researchers working independently of each other around the world found evidence of

mycoplasmas or immune response to them in 30–50% of the rheumatoid arthritis patients tested.[29–38]

- In 1992, Dr. Katherine Ginsburg and her colleagues found that 63% of the female SLE patients they tested had mycoplasmas in their genital membranes. She also reported that specific strains of mycoplasma gave rise to immune responses similar to those seen in lupus.[39]

GERMS ON TRIAL

Before declaring that a disease is caused by microbes, scientists need to identify the responsible germs. Lyme disease presents a very good example of the difficulty in detecting microbial villains after they have "gone underground." It took years for experts in microbial pathology to identify the spirochete microbe that causes Lyme disease. Mycoplasmas and L-form bacteria are the greatest challenge, since they can hide in connective tissues and inside or on the surfaces of immune and other cells. Soon after entering the body, mycoplasmas and L-form bacteria become difficult to detect, except by hi-tech procedures (e.g., polymerase chain reaction, electrophoresis, protein fractionation) that were unavailable until fairly recently.[40, 41] Even the Arthritis Foundation, which has historically been hostile to microbe theory and antibiotic therapy, admits the problem: "Rheumatic diseases, such as rheumatoid arthritis, could result from infections that had occured years earlier. . . . It would explain the difficulty of isolating an infectious agent from persons with rheumatoid arthritis, for by the time the arthritis has developed, it may be too late to recover the agent."[42]

Doctors can try to confirm the presence of mycoplasmas and L-form bacteria by identifying specific antibodies that the body creates to attack them. The antibodies to these elusive microbes, however, appear and then vanish from the blood in a cyclical pattern, making detection a hit-or-miss proposition. These variations in antibody levels provide indirect evidence of a bacterial infection, because they resemble the fluctuations in symptoms and blood tests seen in brucellosis (undulant fever) and rheumatoid arthritis. (Brucellosis is a bovine and human disease caused by a bacterium that mutates into L-forms that resemble mycoplasmas.)

Detection can also be frustrated by the fact that the microbes may be hidden in immune complexes. In fact, standard laboratory tests cannot reliably reveal the presence of mycoplasmas hidden in cells, joint tissues, or immune complexes, yet these are the very places mycoplasmas and L-form bacteria hide when attacked by the body's immune system.[43, 44] There is one more clue which rheumatic diseases may be triggered by microbes. The autoimmune attacks in rheumatic diseases are typically led by special TH1 cells, which the body uses to lead the fight against microbes that have burrowed deep inside cells and tissue structures—as mycoplasmas and viruses often do. Moreover, TH1-directed attacks on microbes often result in the kind of tissue damage seen in rheumatoid arthritis.[45]

ANTIBIOTIC THERAPY

During the half-century when microbe theory and antibiotic therapy were left to wander in the medical wilderness, Dr. Brown and a few colleagues were documenting great successes in relieving rheumatic symptoms with antibiotics. Published summaries of the contents of Dr. Brown's vast case files provided persuasive but scientifically inconclusive evidence to support the efficacy of his work.[46] New clinical trials were needed to prove the value of antibiotic therapy. And the value seems high, based on the results of highly credible trials conducted during the first half of the 1990s—and an exciting study published in 1997.

ANTIBIOTIC THERAPY
BOOSTED BY MIRA TRIAL

Antibiotic therapy gained new attention in the early 1990s, when well-controlled clinical trials in Holland and Israel showed that minocycline, a form of tetracycline, was effective against rheumatoid arthritis.[47-50] It earned even more credibility in 1995, with publication of the Minocycline in Rheumatoid Arthritis (MIRA) clinical trial—a well-designed American study sponsored by the NIH. Its highly credible findings indicate that over the course of one year, the antibiotic drugs tetracycline and minocycline are at least as effective as other rheumatoid arthritis drugs and much safer.

The MIRA results also provide more evidence that microbes can cause rheumatic diseases. As Dr. Harold Paulus of the University of California at Los Angeles put it in the editorial accompanying the MIRA report, "The improvement [in blood measures of disease activity] . . . resembles that seen with treatment of a smoldering chronic infection. . . . This suggests that a well-protected infection may be at least partially responsible for rheumatoid arthritis. . . . An intracellular infection that is partially protected from the administered antibiotic agents (for example, *Mycoplasma* infection) might fit the clinical observations."[51]

MIRA RESULTS: EVEN BETTER THAN REPORTED

What exactly did the MIRA trial show? Over forty-eight weeks, 219 adults with mild to moderate rheumatoid arthritis received either minocycline or a placebo. At the end of the trial period, the minocycline group showed greater improvement in joint tenderness (54% versus 39%), joint swelling (54% versus 41%), and blood measures of disease activity. The authors concluded that "minocycline was safe and effective for patients with mild to moderate rheumatoid arthritis. Its mechanisms of action remain to be determined."[52]

If anything, this conclusion understates the case, since the minocycline group experienced much better symptomatic relief than the final numbers suggest. As the MIRA authors wrote, "Several factors may have contributed to this [greater than expected improvement in the placebo group] . . . and may have minimized the differences in outcomes." The authors were alluding to the fact that many in the placebo group violated the rules by receiving steroids, SAARDs, or greater amounts of NSAIDs than allowed, while many in the minocycline group actually lowered their intake of NSAIDs. A respected expert in experimental statistics later critiqued the authors' conclusions as being too conservative in light of the facts: "This [statistical] bias obscures the superiority of the minocycline treatment over the placebo in reducing joint pain and swelling."[53]

Together with similar results seen in foreign trials, the results of the landmark MIRA study establish four important facts. First, compared with a placebo (sugar pill), minocycline gives significantly better symptomatic relief and improvements in laboratory measures of disease activity. Second, minocycline has fewer and milder side effects (stomach upset or dizziness) than steroids, SAARDs, or cytotoxic drugs. Third, minocycline therapy leads patients to spontaneously limit the use of other drugs (NSAIDs, SAARDs, steroids). And, last, minocycline produces increasing symptomatic relief over time; improvement lasts for weeks after the drug is discontinued.

NEW PROOF OF ANTIBIOTIC THERAPY

In 1997, Dr. James O'Dell presented an exciting scientific study to the American College of Rheumatology conference in Washington, D.C. As the Associated Press reported, the audience's reaction was enthusiastic. "Rheumatologists said the new study by the University of Nebraska provides enough proof of minocycline's benefit that the drug soon may be widely prescribed." Considering that no new drugs for rheumatoid arthritis have been found in decades, this is quite a vindication of Tom Brown's career. Dr. O'Dell claimed no cure in his report, saying that "if the medicine is stopped the problem comes back." On the other hand, the study lasted only six months and employed fairly modest doses of antibiotic (200 milligrams per day vs. the 400 milligrams often prescribed). The rather short duration of the study is key, because it has been established that patients receiving this therapy continue to improve over time.

How can we account for the superior results achieved by Dr. O'Dell's team? Remember that in the MIRA trial, which included many cases of long duration, many in the placebo group continued to take antirheumatic drugs and NSAIDs. In O'Dell's trial, patients had had the disease for less than one year, and few subjects were on second-line drug therapy. The objective was to determine whether minocycline is an effective therapy for seropositive rheumatoid arthritis when used within the first year of disease. The Rheumatoid Arthritis Investigational Network enrolled forty-six patients with rheumatoid arthritis of less than one year's duration. All patients were rheumatoid factor positive. After six months, 65% of the minocycline group met the authors' "50% improvement" criteria versus only 13% of the placebo group—a statistically significant result.[54]

ANTIBIOTICS AS ANTI-INFLAMMATORY DRUGS

The positive results of the various clinical trials of antibiotic therapy may mean one or both of two things: 1) We are close to a cure for some cases of rheumatoid arthritis; 2) Tetracycline-type antibiotics alleviate symptoms more safely and durably than conventional antirheumatic drugs. It is likely that at least some of the benefits of antibiotic therapy have nothing to do with microbes, because tetracycline-type drugs have several important properties.

Tetracycline drugs strongly inhibit the action of enzymes (collagenase, metalloproteinase, etc.) believed to destroy collagen during inflammatory episodes.[55, 56] In particular, minocycline appears to chelate (bind to) calcium, thereby preventing release of collagenase from cells.[57] As Dr. O'Dell said in his 1997 presentation to the American College of Rheumatology, "By inhibiting these metalloproteinases early on, maybe we can shut off the whole inflammation cascade."

Moreover, tetracycline-type antibiotics are potent anti-inflammatory agents and also suppress damaging immune responses by T cells.[58–60]

SIDE EFFECTS OF ANTIBIOTICS

Lest you take away an excessively rosy picture of antibiotic therapy, it is important to note that antibiotics are toxic substances that are accompanied by undesirable side effects:

- Antibiotics destroy beneficial *Lactobacillus* bacteria that colonize human intestines. These immune-supportive microbes produce vitamins, promote efficient digestion, and help keep disease microbes—including stubborn yeasts such as *Candida albicans*—in check. Beneficial intestinal bacteria can be restored by eating yogurt containing live *S. thermophilus* and *L. bulgaricus* cultures (any yogurt bearing the industry's voluntary "live cultures" seal) or by taking dietary supplements of beneficial *Lactobacillus* cultures (*L. acidophilus*, *L. bifidus*, etc.).
- Antibiotics can promote leaky gut syndrome, which might aggravate rheumatic inflammations. Given the clinical results, however, this appears to be a minor concern.
- Tetracycline and its derivative drugs can cause other, minor side effects, including nausea, sensitivity to sunlight, and rashes.
- Use of antibiotics encourages the growth of strains of resistant bacteria. Tetracycline-class antibiotics like minocycline are less likely to do this because of the way they attack microbes.
- One aspect of antibiotic therapy that patients must be prepared for is the Jarisch-Herxheimer reaction—a temporary worsening of symptoms that accompanies the release of toxins by dying microbes. This positive sign of antimicrobial effect should recede within several weeks or with temporary reductions in dosage.

ARE ANTIBIOTICS RIGHT FOR YOU?

Before moving to antibiotics, it makes sense to try a medically supervised therapeutic plan that combines dietary changes, therapeutic supplements (vitamins, nutraceuticals, herbs), physical therapy, and various mind–body techniques, including acupuncture, guided imagery, and biofeedback (see Chapter 9). If this "natural" approach fails to lead to significant improvement, you should consider drug therapies that can minimize the risk of joint damage. The point at which this decision becomes critical is best determined in consultation with a rheumatologist or an internist with comparable experience and training. Many people may be able to rely on natural therapies indefinitely, if regular laboratory tests show that this approach is controlling inflammations well enough to prevent joint damage. If not, antibiotics seem to be a safer, fundamentally more germane choice than gold and other rheumatoid arthritis drugs. To the extent that microbes are triggering your symptoms, antibiotics could be far more effective over the long term.

ANTIBIOTIC THERAPY: INFORMATION RESOURCES

Few medical doctors are familiar with antibiotic therapy for rheumatic diseases. Dr. Brown used various antibiotics—primarily tetracycline and minocycline but also doxycycline, linomycin, cleocin, vibramycin, erythromycin, ampicillin, and amoxicillin. The tetracycline-class drugs work especially well against mycoplasmas. Other antibiotics are more useful against streptococci, salmonellae, and the various bacteria that can cause rheumatic conditions.

The antibiotic regimen for rheumatic diseases differs significantly from standard therapy for infectious diseases in terms of both dosage and schedule. Patients and colleagues of Dr. Brown established a resource group called The Road Back Foundation, which provides information for physicians about proper use of antibiotics for rheumatic diseases (see "Antibiotic Therapy" in Appendix A). The foundation also offers information and support to patients. Patients or physicians interested in antibiotic therapy should also read *The Arthritis Breakthrough*, an excellent history of microbe theory and antibiotic therapy listed in the bibliography.

CHAPTER 15

HOMEOPATHIC REMEDIES

IN 1980, the *British Journal of Clinical Pharmacology* published a controlled, double-blind clinical study of an unusual arthritis remedy. Nothing about it was unusual except that the experimental remedy contained no detectable medicine—just sugar. Yet the researchers reported that 82% of participants given the "homeopathic" remedies experienced relief versus only 21% of those receiving placebo pills that were equally devoid of chemicals other than sugar.[1] A second British study, published in 1983, found no difference between two sugar pills —one used as a placebo and one containing the homeopathic remedy called Rhus tox. 6X.[2] What made the crucial difference between the two sets of sugar pills in the first study? Is there other evidence that homeopathy may work? Proponents say that homeopathic remedies contain the invisible, energetic imprints of natural substances that prompt helpful healing responses. The story behind the confounding mystery of homeopathy is certainly colorful.

In the late 1600s, Jesuit priests in South America observed that Indians native to the Amazon who were sent into cold, damp Spanish mines would alleviate their chills and shivering by drinking a tea made from the bark of the chincona tree. The Jesuits conceived the idea that chincona might work on fevers, and within a few years "Jesuit's powder" had swept Europe as a cure for malaria. Today this remarkable herbal remedy is prescribed in the form of a synthetic drug called quinine. Taken in large amounts, chincona bark and quinine both engender symptoms very like those of malaria. And it was this serendipitous discovery that later inspired the founder of homeopathy.

The basic theory behind homeopathy—"like cures like"—dates back to Hippocrates, but it was a German doctor named Samuel Hahnemann (1755–1843) who developed the practice of homeopathy. Intrigued by the example of quinine and malaria, Hahnemann decided to see whether other medicines could be made from substances that produced the symptoms of the disease they were intended to cure. First, he observed the symptoms produced in volunteers by various plant, mineral, and animal substances. Hahnemann then diluted each substance to the extreme and tested the resulting "homeopathic remedy" against diseases known to have similar symptoms. Hahnemann called this principle of prescription the Law of Similars and proposed that the remedies work by stimulating the body to respond to the threats they mimic. The common remedy called allium cepa (onion) offers a good example. Like the allergens that give rise to hay fever, fumes from a cut onion will provoke red, teary eyes and runny noses. An extremely dilute solution of onion was tested by early homeopaths and declared to be an effective remedy for hay fever symptoms.

Hahnemann and several German colleagues conducted hundreds of these uncontrolled clinical trials—a semiscientific approach that put them well ahead of their time. The results were compiled in a series of "materia medica," or directories, matching homeopathic remedies to disease conditions and various combinations of personal characteristics. Hahnemann's research had led him to believe that a homeopathic prescription needed to take into account the patient's physical, mental, and emotional characteristics as well as their symptoms.

By the 1850s, Hahnemann's theory was embraced by many mainstream physicians, and homeopathic medical schools numbered in the hundreds. Homeopathy gained a strong boost in the United States following serious cholera and yellow fever epidemics in the 1830s. Patients who received homeopathic treatment were widely reported to have recovered in much greater numbers than patients who received the limited, decidedly nonscientific medical treatments then available.

LESS IS MORE, AD INFINITUM: THE PARADOX OF HOMEOPATHY

Medical science completely rejects the hypothesis that lies at the core of homeopathy—namely, that the potency of homeopathic remedies increases as the dose decreases. The remedies are prepared by making successive dilutions of the original substance in water or alcohol, and the weaker the dilution, the stronger the healing effect. Skeptics point out that most homeopathic remedies are so dilute that they do not contain even a single molecule of the original substance. Proponents believe that homeopathic remedies contain some sort of energetic imprint of the original substance, which subtly influences the body— or a bio-energetic field within it—in ways as yet unknown to science. In the late 1980s, French physicists claimed to have produced laboratory evidence of such energetic imprints, but these results remain unaccepted by most of their scientific colleagues.

THE RETURN OF HOMEOPATHY

To many physicians of the early nineteenth century, homeopathy seemed more credible and scientific than the dangerously crude therapies and surgical methods of the day. They had good reason to embrace this new theory, supported as it was by the results of hundreds of rudimentary clinical experiments. Homeopathy lost ground at the turn of the century, as surgeons refined their skills and chemists made better drugs. And as physicists discovered more about the nature of matter and energy, the principle of inverse potency was mocked as utterly implausible. By 1900, homeopathy had nearly been driven out of existence by competition with new technologies and persecution by the American Medical Association.

In recent years, growing disenchantment with conventional medicine has led to a renaissance of homeopathy. It never lost popularity in India, where there are millions of practitioners and patients. And it has come back strongly in Europe; one in three physicians in France and England prescribes homeopathic remedies—usually for self-correcting complaints such as earaches or hay fever. A few hundred holistic medical doctors in America have added homeopathy to their arsenal of therapies. And thanks to a quirk of U.S. law, makers of homeopathic remedies enjoy the right to make specific therapeutic claims—a privilege denied even to makers of herbal medicines whose safety and efficacy is supported by strong clinical evidence.

DOES IT WORK?

There is a small body of evidence indicating that homeopathic remedies can sometimes produce benefit unexplained by the placebo effect. In 1991, the leading British medical journal *The Lancet* published the results of an analysis of the quality and results of 107 clinical trials of homeopathy. The authors' analysis suggests that the beneficial effect of homeopathy is far from established, but it cannot be rejected out of hand. In 1994, *The Lancet* published the results of a well-controlled clinical study of homeopathy for asthma that was done, as the editors said, "with exceptional rigor." Similarly positive results against influenza made a homeopathic product called Oscillococcinum the best-selling flu remedy in France—a popularity that seems to persist on the basis of users' positive experiences. Reputable practitioners will be the first to emphasize that homeopathy is not appropriate as an exclusive treatment for diseases that can lead to serious injury or death—such as certain types and cases of arthritis. But if used under medical supervision, homeopathy cannot harm the patient—especially as an adjunct to pharmaceutical or nutritional treatment of uncomfortable symptoms.

HOMEOPATHY IN ARTHRITIS

Companies that make homeopathic remedies have vastly increased sales in health stores and drugstores by marketing them like standard drugs. That is, one remedy or combination of remedies is indicated for each condition. But if you want to give homeopathy a serious trial, it makes sense to follow traditional practice and seek out a trained, experienced homeopathic practitioner—ideally a medical doctor—who will prescribe a remedy based on your personal characteristics and symptoms. This kind of customization is considered especially important in the treatment of more serious health conditions. In his book *The Family Guide to Homeopathy*, noted French homeopath Alain Horvilleur, M.D., cautions that "rheumatoid arthritis [and like conditions] should be diagnosed and treated by a medical doctor or rheumatologist." With this strong caveat in mind, here are some of the remedies commonly recommended for specific rheumatic conditions (letters and numbers, such as "12 C," indicate potency/dilution).

- Ankylosing spondylitis: Tuberculinum nosode, 12 C (only in the early stages of the disease)
- Fibromyalgia: Cimicifuga racemosa, 9 C
- Rheumatoid arthritis: Streptococcin nosode, 12 C (only in the early stages of the disease)
- Rheumatic joints: Apis mellifica, 9 C (for painless swelling)
- Rheumatic joints: Bryonia alba, 9 C (for painful swelling)

CHAPTER 16

FOLK REMEDIES

SIR WILLIAM OSLER, FIRST CHIEF OF THE Johns Hopkins Medical School, made this refreshingly frank admission at the close of the nineteenth century: "When a patient with arthritis walks in the front door, I feel like leaving out the back door." There is little wonder Sir William felt this way, since contemporary medical doctors still bemoan the lack of consistently effective remedies for arthritis. (We have reviewed many possibilities they overlook!) Patients of Osler's day turned to herbs and folk medicines—and many modern Americans still do. To narrow your search for effective aids, it will help to examine some of the most famous folk "cures."

ALFALFA
(*MEDICAGO SATIVA* / LUCERNE)
NO EVIDENCE AVAILABLE • SHORT HISTORY • RAISES LUPUS RISK

Alfalfa's folk reputation as an antirheumatic drug seems to be of very recent origin. According to Varro Tyler, Ph.D., America's renowned scientific authority on plant drugs, there are no references to any antirheumatic effects of alfalfa before the early twentieth century. By itself, this is reason for skepticism, since humans have been eating alfalfa and its seed sprouts for thousands of years. It seems that any antirheumatic effects of alfalfa would have been noted and recorded in one of the many herbal pharmacopoeias printed over the past four hundred years. Daniel Mowrey's *Herbal Tonic Therapies* (see Bibliography) states that there is evidence that alfalfa produces antirheumatic benefits in 10–20% of patients. While the author cites several studies, none appear to be relevant to establishing a therapeutic benefit in arthritis.

TOXIC EFFECTS OF ALFALFA

When consumed in large quantities, alfalfa seeds and sprouts trigger SLE in monkeys and aggravate it in people.[1, 2] Small amounts are considered harmless, except for those who have had lupus or may be susceptible to it.

BEE VENOM

LONG TRADITION • SOME POSITIVE EVIDENCE • RESEARCH IN PROGRESS

Use of bee venom, or "apitherapy," for arthritis dates back many centuries. According to the American Apitherapy Association, some three hundred doctors in the United States use it, primarily to treat inflammatory autoimmune disorders. Bee venom can be administered by injection or by holding bees against the skin with tweezers and waiting for the sting. Scientists have begun to research bee venom's potential for treating multiple sclerosis and rheumatic diseases. (Like the rheumatic diseases, multiple sclerosis is an autoimmune condition, but it differs in that it affects the myelin sheath around nerves.) The National Multiple Sclerosis Society does not endorse bee venom therapy, and most researchers characterize it as an unpleasant last resort. Quite a few sufferers, however, claim strong relief—anecdotal evidence that should not be dismissed. According to the *Alternative Medicine Digest*, some 1,500 studies on bee venom are said to have been conducted in Europe and Asia. (The main U.S. medical databases contain none, suggesting that these studies were mostly unpublished or appeared in relatively obscure journals.)

Researchers at the Walter Reed Army Institute of Research found that bee venom contains an anti-inflammatory chemical one thousand times stronger than indomethacin (a potent NSAID) and two chemicals that stimulate release of cortisol. At the Walter Reed Medical Hospital, injections of bee venom gave consistently positive results in dogs with rheumatic diseases. New Jersey-based pain researcher Dr. Christopher Kim conducted a study in which 180 patients with arthritis and related diseases were injected with either bee venom or a placebo; the bee venom group enjoyed better pain relief. Related animal studies are currently under way at the Neurology Department of Thomas Jefferson University in Philadelphia.

Beekeeper Charles Mraz of Middlebury, Vermont, is famous for providing bee stings to arthritis sufferers who request them. Mr. Mraz cautions that those who have claimed major relief have usually achieved it only after receiving thousands of controlled stings over a period of a year or more. To try apitherapy, contact the American Apitherapy Society (see "Bee Venom Therapy" in Appendix A). WARNING: One in every fifty persons is deadly allergic to bee venom. You must be tested in a doctor's office, with antidote on hand, before trying any "sting cure."

COPPER BRACELETS

LONG TRADITION • NO CLINICAL EVIDENCE

Copper wrist bracelets are one of the best-known folk remedies for inflammatory types of arthritis. For decades, doctors have decried them as a waste of money. There is no scientific evidence that arthritis patients benefit from wearing copper, but anecdotal endorsements abound. As noted in Chapter 11, it does make sense to take dietary supplements of copper to maintain general health and for its possible, but unproved, anti-inflammatory effects. Given their low cost and long folk history, it cannot hurt to try copper bracelets, too.

HONEY AND VINEGAR

RECENT TRADITION • NO CLINICAL EVIDENCE

In 1960, Vermont country doctor D. C. Jarvis, M.D., wrote a book entitled *Arthritis and Folk Medicine,* which spread the belief that eating honey and vinegar can help alleviate arthritis. One secondhand anecdotal account relayed to us reported a dramatic cure following repeated immersion of the sufferer's arthritic hands in vinegar. There is no scientific evidence that either food works and no known reason they should. Still, the many anecdotal endorsements in the record suggest that honey and vinegar may work for some, and experimentation is both safe and savory.

RESOURCES

ACUPUNCTURE/ACUPRESSURE/ CHINESE HERBAL MEDICINE

The best referrals are often obtained by word of mouth, but you may also be able to find a good practitioner by contacting an acupuncture association or accredited acupuncture school.

The Council of Colleges of Acupuncture and Oriental Medicine is America's only accrediting body, with twenty-seven member institutions. CCAOM, 8403 Colesville Rd., Suite 370, Silver Springs, MD 20910. Telephone: 301–608–9175. Web site: www.ccaom.org

The National Certification Commission for Acupuncture can refer you to state licensing agencies or to someone the Commission has certified. Telephone: 703-548-9004.

The American Academy of Medical Acupuncture refers callers to medical doctors with acupuncture training. Telephone: 800–521–2262.

For information and referrals, contact the Acupressure Institute, 1533 Shattuck Ave., Berkeley, CA 94709. Telephone: 510–845–1059 inside California, 800-442-2232 outside California. Web site: www.acupressure.com

ANTIBIOTIC THERAPY

The Road Back Foundation, 4985 N. Lake Mill Road, Delaware, OH 43015-9249. Telephone: 740–881–5601.

ASSISTIVE DEVICES

ABLEDATA is a database with information on fifteen thousand disability products. Call 800–344–5405 (203–667–5405 in Connecticut), or write to ABLEDATA, Adaptive Equipment Center, Newington Children's Hospital, 181 E. Cedar St., Newington, CT 06111. Web site: www.abledata.com

BEE VENOM THERAPY

American Apitherapy Society, P.O. Box 54, Hartland Four Corners, VT 05049. Telephone: 802–436-2708.

BOVINE CARTILAGE

Vitacarte, from Phoenix Bio Logic, 1117 E. Putnam Ave., Suite 242, Riverside, CT 06878. Telephone: 800–947-8482. Web site: www.vicarte.com

BiocartilageÆ, from Biocar Laboratories Ltd., Division of Lescarden, Inc., Suite 2025, 420 Lexington Ave., New York, NY 10170. Telephone: 212–687–1050. Web site: www.lescarden.com

CONVENTIONAL CARE AND COPING STRATEGIES

For information and referrals, contact the Arthritis Foundation, 1314 Spring Street NW, Atlanta, GA 30309. Telephone: 800–283–7800. Web site: www.arthritis.org

CHINESE HERBAL MEDICINE

GENERAL INFORMATION

The American Association of Oriental Medicine, 433 Front St., Catasqua, PA 18032. Telephone: 610–433–2448. Web site: www.aaom.org

The Web That Has No Weaver, by Ted Kaptchuk, may be the best Western guide to the theory and practice of Chinese traditional medicine. The book will be reprinted in 1999 in a Fifteenth Anniversary Edition. It can be ordered through Amazon.com under the title *The Web That Has No Weaver: Understanding Chinese Medicine*.

SPECIFIC INFORMATION

Oriental Materia Medica: A Concise Guide by Hong-Yen Hsu, et al. Available from the American Botanical Council catalog as item no. B157. Call 800–373–7105 or fax your request to 512–331–1924. The council's bookstore also has several other versions of the Chinese Materia Medica. Web sites: www.herbalgram.org, www.herbalgram.org/catalog/asia.html

Pharmacology and Applications of Chinese Materia Medica, vol. 2, by the Chinese Medicinal Material Research Centre, the Chinese University of Hong Kong (World Scientific Publishers). Web site: www.worldscientific.com

DIETARY SUPPLEMENTS

Health food stores carry the best selection of "natural" vitamins, herbs, and nutraceutical products—which means that they are relatively free of artificial additives and common allergens. Some pharmacies also offer a respectable range of the more common products and natural brands. Several Web sites offer a large selection together with a good amount of fairly objective information, including: www.mothernature.com, www.greentree.com, www.vitaminshoppe.com, and www.healthshop.com.

If you have difficulty finding a retail outlet near you, call the National Nutritional Foods Association at 714–622–6272. They may be able to supply a list of manufacturers who sell by mail order. If not, you can request the toll-free telephone numbers for the following brands, which are recognized for reliable quality:

VITAMINS AND NUTRACEUTICALS

Country Life, Enzymatic Therapy, FutureBiotics, GNC, Health from the Sun (especially for GLA), KAL, Nature's Way (especially for OPC), Solgar, Sundown (Rexall), Schiff, Thompson, and Twin Lab.

HERBAL PRODUCTS

Gaia Herbs, Herb Pharm, East Earth Herbs, Nature's Herbs, Nature's Way, Pure World (for Kava), Rainbow Light, and Zand.

EMU OIL

Emu Man Direct, 408 Columbia St. no. 207, Hood River, Oregon 97031. Telephone: 800–315–3687.

Old Well Corporation, PO Box 19351, Raleigh, NC 27619. Telephone: 800–269–0506.

FELDENKRAIS

For information and referrals, contact the Feldenkrais Guild, P.O. Box 489, Albany, OR 97321. Telephone: 503–926–0981. Web site: www.feldenkrais.com

FIBROMYALGIA

For a free information packet, send a stamped, self-addressed envelope to the National Fibromyalgia Research Association, P.O. Box 500, Salem, OR 97308. The association also offers a video on proper exercise at a cost of $24.95.

GUIDED IMAGERY

For referrals, contact the Academy for Guided Imagery, P.O. Box 2070, Mill Valley, CA 94942. Telephone: 800–726–2070.

HEMP SEED OIL

The Ohio Hempery, 7002 S.R. 329, Guysville, OH 45735. Telephone: 800–289–4367 or 614–662–4367. Web site: www.hempery.com

HERB INFORMATION

American Botanical Council. Web site: www.herbalgram.org

HOMEOPATHY

For a catalog of products, educational materials, and resources, contact Homeopathic Educational Services, 2124 Kittredge St., Berkeley, CA 94704. Telephone: 510–649–0294. Web site: www.homeopathic.com

For information and referrals, contact the International Foundation for Homeopathy, 2366 Eastlake Ave. East, no. 301, Seattle, WA 98102; or the National Center for Homeopathy, 801 N. Fairfax, Suite 306, Alexandria, VA 22314. Telephone: 703–548–7790.

NATUROPATHIC PHYSICIANS

For referrals, contact the American Association of Naturopathic Physicians, 2366 Eastlake Ave., Suite 322, Seattle, WA 98102. Telephone: 206–298–0125. Web site: www.naturopathic.org

Or contact one of two U.S. Department of Education accredited naturopathic colleges for referrals.

Bastyr University, 144 NE 54th St., Seattle, WA 98105. Telephone: 206–523–9585. Web site: www.bastyr.edu/alumni/

National College of Naturopathic Medicine, 049 SW Porter, Portland, OR 97201. Web site: www.ncnm.edu/sap.htm

NEUROMUSCULAR THERAPISTS

Check your Yellow Pages for NMT practitioners listed under Massage and inquire as to their training in NMT. I have had good personal experience with licensed massage therapists who are certified in the St. John method of neuromuscular therapy.

PAIN MANAGEMENT / RELAXATION

Arthritis Self-Management Program. Call the National Arthritis Foundation at 800–283–7800. Web site: www.arthritis.org

Cognitive Behavioral Therapy. For a referral to a CBT specialist near you, send a request to the Association for Advancement of Behavioral Therapy, 305 7th Ave., New York, NY 10001. Include a $5.00 check or money order to cover postage and handling. Telephone: 212–647–1890. Web site: www.aabt.org/aabt

PHYSICAL THERAPISTS

Call your county or state medical society for the local branch of the American Physical Therapy Association.

The Cybex Medical Device Corp. also maintains a list. Telephone: 800–222–3245.

ROLFING

For information and referrals, contact the International Rolf Institute, P.O. Box 1868, Boulder, CO 80306. Telephone: 303–449–5903. Web site: www.rolf.org

THERAPEUTIC EXERCISE

The Arthritis Foundation recommends a program called PACE. Contact your local foundation office by getting its telephone number from the national office at 800-722-5236. Web site: www.arthritis.org.

MORE HERBAL OPTIONS

KEY TO ABBREVIATIONS

AA = antianxiety

AB = antibacterial

AH = antihistamine

AI = anti-inflammatory

AN = analgesic

AS = adrenal support

AV = antiviral

AX = antioxidant

DI = diuretic

HS = hepatic (liver) support

IM = immune-modulating

MR = muscle relaxant

TCM = traditional Chinese medicine

TN = temperature normalization

HERBS AND BOTANICAL EXTRACTS

The herbs covered in Chapter 12 are supported by either positive clinical evidence or a particularly strong tradition of folk use in arthritis. They are not the only options. There are many other single herbs and Chinese herbal formulas that may be just as effective in your case. Herbs are included here if they meet one or both of two criteria: there is reasonable scientific evidence for safety and relevant physiological effects and/or a significant tradition of medicinal use in arthritis or related conditions.

Consult with a physician and trained, experienced herbalist or licensed acupuncturist before using any of these herbs. Note: Long-term use of whole licorice extract at high doses can cause hypertension. Chronic use of sarsaparilla at high doses can cause temporary kidney impairment and increase absorption of digitalis.

CHINESE PATENT MEDICINES

These Chinese patent medicines have had long histories of use for various types of arthritis. They are normally prescribed by practitioners trained in traditional Chinese medicine, to complement and enhance acupuncture treatment. While their efficacy has probably not been subjected to clinical testing, they have stood the test of time. The last remedy mentioned is an American product based on classic Chinese theory, which describes arthritis as a condition of "cold, wind, and damp" that interferes with the meridian system that outlines the periphery of the body.

CHIN KOO TIEH SHANG WAN
Tientsin Drug Manufacturing, Tientsin, China

This remedy is labeled for traumatic injury, dislocation of joints, sprains, and strains. The pills are said to alleviate inflammation, swelling, and pain and may therefore help lessen the risk of chronic arthritis stemming from trauma to joints. This medicine contains pseudoginseng root, dragon blood resin, dong guai *(Angelica sinensis)*, frankincense *(Boswellia serrata)* resin, myrrh *(commiphora mukul)* resin, and carthamus flower.

Frankincense and myrrh have proven anti-inflammatory and analgesic properties. *Carthamus tinctorius* is a proven anticoagulant herb. *Angelica sinensis* is a proven muscle relaxant and may be an anti-inflammatory. Caution: carthamus and angelica are contraindicated during pregnancy.

Folk and Botanical Name	Relevant Effects and Traditions
Ashwaganda root/leaf (*Withania somnifera*)	AI•Indian (Ayurvedic) herb for arthritis
Astragalus/Huangqi root (*Astragalus membranaceus*)	IM•TCM for immune support
Cangzhu rhizome (*Atractolydes lancea*)	AI•AB•AV•TCM for rheumatism
Black Cohosh (*Cimicifuga racemosa*)	AI•TCM and Native American use for rheumatism
Cat's claw/Uña de gato† (*Uncaria tomentosa* or *U. guianensis*)	IM•AI•AX•Amazonian use for rheumatism
Chuchuhuasi† (*Maytenus macrocarpa, M. laevis, M. ebenifolia,* or *M. krukovii*)	IM•AI•AX•Amazonian use for rheumatism
Epimedium leaf/twig (*Epimedium brevicornum*)	AI•IM•TCM for rheumatism
Elder root/twigs (*Sambucus williamsii, S. canadensis, S. nigra*)	AV•TCM for rheumatism
Fang Feng Root (*Saposhnikovia divaricata*)	AI•AN•TCM for rheumatism
Ganoderma/Reishi/Lingzhi (*Ganoderma lucidum*)	AI•TCM for joints, tendons, bones
Gentian rhizomes/root (*Gentian lutea*)	AI • TCM for rheumatoid arthritis
Giant knotweed/Huzhang (*Polygonum caspidatum*)	AI•AX•AV•AB•AH•TCM for rheumatism
Kava root (*Piper methysticum*)	AN•MR•AA•Oceanic traditional use for arthritis
Licorice root/stolon (*Glycyrrhiza glabra* or *G. uralensis*)	AI•HS*•AA•Enhances corticosteroid activity •TCM for rheumatism
Gaoben roots and rhizome (*Ligusticum sinense,* etc.)	AI•AN•AH•TCM for rheumatism
Luffa (loofah) vine fruit (*Luffa cylindrica,* etc.)	AI•AN•TCM for inflammation
Milk thistle/silymarin (*Silybum marianum*)	AX•HS
Picrorrizha kurroa root (kahti roots, Picroliv, Apocynin)	AI•IM•HS

Sangre de drago/dragon's blood[†]
(Croton lechleri, C. draconoides,
C. palanostigma, C. erthrochilis)

AI•AX•Amazonian use for pain,
inflammation

Sarsaparilla root and rhizome
(Smilax medica, S. sieboldi, etc.)

AI•AN•HS•TCM use for rheumatism

---

[*]Licorice is contraindicated for people with hypertension (unless it is in a deglycyrrhizinated form), or cholestatic liver disorders, or cirrhosis, and for women who are pregnant. (Glycyrrhizine is an active compound in licorice that can promote hypertension.)

[†]For a complete review of these three very promising Amazonian herbs, we recommend *Cat's Claw*, by Kenneth Jones (Sylvan Press, 1995)—a well-researched and fully referenced resource. All three—especially Sangre de drago—are high in OPCs.

CORYDALIS YANHUSUS ANALGESIC TABLETS
Chongqing Chinese Medicine Factory, Chongqing Sichuan, China

The label states that it "breaks obstruction of energy and blood" and is "good for chronic pain." It contains corydalis rhizome (66%) and angelica root (34%).

TIN TZAT TO CHUNG
Shan Sai Hang Lam Medicine Manufactory, Hong Kong

The medicine is labeled as "relief for arthritic pains and rheumatisms," and is claimed to enhance "circulation of blood and relieve muscle fatigue, ease swelling in hands and legs, relieve stiffness." It contains *Gynura pinnatifida, Eucommia ulmoides* (du jung), *Panax ginseng, Cervus sika* (deer antler), *Ginnamomum loureiru, Pistacia lentiscus, Loranthus ydoripi, Agalloch,* and *Angelica grosserrata.*

ZHENG GU SHI
Yulin Drug Factory, Kwangsi, China

This medicine is labeled as a "topical liniment for aching joints." It contains pseudoginseng root; croton seed; cinnamon bark, angelica root, alcohol, gentiana qin jao, inula flower, menthol crystal, and camphor crystal.

ARTHRITIC

This is a formula in the "Jade Herbals" line from East Earth Herb Inc., P.O. Box 2802, Eugene, OR 97402. Telephone: 800–827–4372.

The primary actions are to "relieve impaired flexibility, nourish yin, alleviate meridian obstruction." It contains Cortex salicis albae, Cortex Erythinae, Flos Lonicerae, Rhizoma Gastrodiae, Flos Carthami, and Radix Glycyrrhizae.

TOP HERBS: SCIENTIFIC SUMMARIES

BOSWELLIA

The anti-inflammatory effects of boswellia on animals are well proved. Based on the results of three preliminary clinical trials, including one double-blind, placebo-controlled study, boswellic acids rival the anti-inflammatory action of NSAIDs but without the adverse side effects.

BOSWELLIA VERSUS NSAIDs

In one of several similar studies involving rats, boswellic acids were compared with phenylbutazone, a potent synthetic NSAID. Boswellia decreased artificially induced swelling by an average of 57% compared with 47% for phenylbutazone.[1–3] Boswellic acids are effective NSAIDs because they attack inflammation from three angles.

- Unlike aspirin, but like some other NSAIDs, boswellic acids curtail excess production of the most potent inflammatory mediators, called leukotrienes, by interfering with the inflammatory cascade reaction produced by 5-lipoxygenase enzyme. This effect helps explain why boswellic acids do not cause the side effects associated with NSAIDs that block COX-1 and 12-lipoxygenase enzymes.[4, 5]

• Boswellic acids limit the migration of inflammatory immune cells to inflamed tissues.[6, 7]

• Boswellic acids disrupt the inflammatory autoimmune response at earlier stages—specifically primary antibody production and complement (immune protein) activity.[8, 9]

CAN BOSWELLIA PROTECT CARTILAGE?

Over time, the inflammatory pain of rheumatoid arthritis can be joined by pain from the gradual destruction of cartilage caused by secondary osteoarthrosis. Based on animal studies, boswellic acids may help prevent this degradation and pain by minimizing the "leaking" of GAGs from cartilage (see Chapter 4). This critical problem characterizes osteoarthrosis and is a secondary result of rheumatoid inflammations.[10]

CLINICAL TRIALS

To test boswellic acids against rheumatoid arthritis and ankylosing spondylitis, 175 patients who had had little relief from other treatments were given 600 milligrams per day of boswellia extract for at least four weeks. Based on a standard measure of clinical improvement (the Mean Arthritic Score), two of three experienced good to excellent results: 14% had excellent, 53% good, and 30% fair results after four weeks.[11, 12]

In an uncontrolled study by the Medical College of Patiala, India, 30 patients were given 600 milligrams per day of boswellia extract. After four weeks, their average Mean Arthritic Score dropped by

47%, and the ESR—a standard blood measure of disease activity—fell by 36%.[13, 14]

The most reliable results were obtained from a double-blind, placebo-controlled, crossover study of 30 patients who first received either a placebo or 600 milligrams of boswellic acids and then switched over to test the effects of the change. In those receiving boswellic acids, the average Mean Arthritic Score fell by 60% and the ESR dropped by 25%. After switching over to a placebo, the Mean Arthritic Score and ESR rose again, but to lower levels than before.[15]

GINGER

Ginger's therapeutic promise is supported by extensive evidence of strong anti-inflammatory effects in animals and the very positive results of two preliminary clinical trials from Denmark.

CLINICAL TRIALS

In the first study, 7 patients were given ginger for three months, and each of them reported better relief from stiffness, swelling, and pain than they had experienced from synthetic NSAIDs.[16] In the second study, ginger was given to 28 patients with rheumatoid arthritis, 18 patients with osteoarthrosis, and 10 patients with fibromyalgia-like symptoms. In the end, three of four experienced significant relief from pain and swelling.[17]

SHOSAIKOTO (BUPF)

Bupf root contains chemicals called saikosaponins, which possess potent anti-inflammatory properties. The other ingredients in shosaikoto also offer anti-inflammatory effects, produced by various physiological mechanisms.[18–22] Eastern and Western researchers have reported that shosaikoto and related kampo medicines containing licorice are effective against autoimmune disorders in animals.[23] In particular, licorice has been shown to significantly increase the clearance of immune complexes in mice with carageenan-induced rheumatic arthritis.[24]

In addition to other modes of anti-inflammatory action, shosaikoto enhances the effects of corticosteroid drugs, stimulates internal production of cortisols, and protects the adrenal glands from weakening under repeated doses of corticosteroid drugs. These experimental results could be of great significance for patients taking supplemental steroids, since oral shosaikoto might enhance the effectiveness of lower doses while minimizing side effects.[25–27] Shosaikoto also normalizes the function of the immune system. In rats with weakened immune systems, administration of shosaikoto boosted the immune response of macrophage cells. In rats suffering from overactive immune systems, as in rheumatic disorders, the Bupf formula suppressed the excessive immune response.[28–30]

LEI-GONG-TENG

Lei-gong-teng seems to affect two different aspects of the rheumatic disease process. In mice, and in human tissues examined in the test tube, Lei-gong-teng suppresses the actions of various immune cells (lymphocytes and monocytes) key to the autoimmune assault on joint tissues. As one Chinese author concluded, "The results of this trial correlate well with clinical trials, suggesting that the therapeutic effect of TII [T2] is associated with its immunosuppressive activity."[31] American researchers shed more light on the subject when they tested T2 on human immune cells in the test tube. They found that it suppressed key immune cells and their production of disease-aggravating molecules without entirely suppressing their immune function.[32–35]

ANTI-INFLAMMATORY

In rheumatoid arthritis patients, another fraction of Lei-gong-teng, called T4, inhibits the synovial cells' production of the key inflamma-tory mediator PGE_2, although not as strongly as the most potent NSAIDs.[36]

BOOSTS INTERNAL CORTICOSTEROIDS

Like the Shosaikoto formula, Lei-gong-teng seems to enhance the formation and/or potency of anti-inflammatory adrenal steroids in arthritic rats while preventing shrinkage of the adrenal gland. In a test against the steroidal drug prednisone, Lei-gong-teng boosted blood levels of corticosterone and the size of the adrenal gland. In contrast, prednisone (a synthetic steroid) lowered blood levels of corticosterone and the size of the adrenal gland. The authors concluded that "the effect of promoting production of corticosteroids may be one of the mechanisms by which T2 can effectively treat autoimmune diseases."[37]

CLINICAL TRIALS: RHEUMATOID ARTHRITIS AND SLE (LUPUS)

The trials summarized here offer examples of successes seen in a large majority of patients. A significant minority experience temporary adverse effects, but the results of one new study we summarize here (the fourth one) indicate that the side effects of the T2 fraction can be sharply reduced without lessening Lei-gong-teng's unique efficacy.

In an uncontrolled study of 144 rheumatic patients—most with rheumatoid arthritis—91% (132 patients) were judged to have expe-rienced positive results, based on clinical and blood measures of dis-ease activity. Twenty-four, or 17.6%, were found to have had total remission (no symptoms, normal blood measures); fifty-four, or 37.5%, were judged to have experienced effective treatment (less joint pain, normal mobility, normal ESR, no rheumatoid factor); and fifty-four were determined to have shown improvement (less joint pain, better mobility, lower ESR). Quite a few experienced side effects, including poor appetite (20%), dry mouth (18.7%), skin rash (15.9%), skin color changes (13.2%), nausea (6.9%) and menstrual disturbances (23% of women). Two men had temporary breast enlargement. The intestinal disturbances were short-lived and receded within a few days.[38]

The same research team tried Lei-gong-teng on ninety-five patients with rheumatoid arthritis and ankylosing spondylitis over periods ranging from two months to two years. Almost all saw some improvement in joint pain, and about 87% had improvement in swelling as well as pain, with benefits appearing within two weeks. Again, a large minority experienced side effects of a relatively minor, transitory nature. In almost half of menstruating women in the trial, there was a cessation or a change in the menstrual cycle that lasted until the herbal drug was discontinued.[39]

At the end of a four-month Chinese trial that enlisted seventy rheumatoid arthritis patients, the authors wrote, "An impressive curative effect of T2 is confirmed much more convincingly by the present study than by the previously reported clinical open [uncontrolled] trials." Compared with the controls taking a placebo, the patients receiving T2 improved in most clinical and blood measures of disease activity after a month of treatment. When the T2 group was secretly switched over to a placebo for the last four weeks, the benefits continued strongly, in some cases for months.

As with synthetic SAARDs, however, almost one in four patients taking T2 for over one month dropped out owing to the side effects, all of which disappeared after discontinuing the drug. These effects were not judged life-threatening, but the patients clearly found them unacceptable in comparison with their disease symptoms.[40]

This trial was repeated, using a lower dose of T2. Equal benefits were documented in 32 rheumatoid arthritis patients, and there were significantly fewer side effects.[41]

Of 26 SLE patients treated with the root and stems (30–60 grams) of Lei-gong-teng, 24 experienced fair to excellent results after 14 days.

- Eight patients enjoyed clinical remission (all skin lesions in remission).
- Ten patients showed "marked improvement" (more than half of lesions in remission).
- Six had some regression of lesions.

Side effects were relatively minor, and five months of follow-up revealed no lasting toxicity.[42]

Of 103 SLE patients treated with the root and stems (30–45 grams) of Lei-gong-teng, 94 were determined to be "improved" or "markedly improved" after 30 days.

- Fifty-six showed marked improvement in symptoms, blood measures, or the ability to limit or stop corticosteroid therapy.
- Lupus cell test results became negative in 23 of 103 subjects, rheumatoid factor disappeared in 75.9%, titer measurement for positive antinuclear antibodies decreased in 29 of 66 subjects, and complement (immune protein) increased or normalized in 19 of 21 subjects who had low levels before treatment.

Side effects, most minor and transitory, were similar to those seen in other trials. One-third of menstruating women experiencing cycle upsets found they resolved within two to six months after treatment stopped.[43]

DEVIL'S CLAW ROOT

Several animal studies testing devil's claw against the NSAID called indomethacin showed fair to good anti-inflammatory and analgesic effects, but they involved abdominal injections of whole herb extract.[44, 45] In contrast, animal studies using oral doses have failed to show significant results, suggesting that the plant's anti-inflammatory components—which remain unknown—cannot survive the digestive process.[46] Because devil's claw exerts fairly strong anti-inflammatory effects when injected into the skin or muscle near joints, it may be a safe alternative to steroids for treating episodes of extreme joint pain. Injectable extracts of devil's claw are available from the German pharmaceutical companies DHU and Hagen.

CLINICAL TRIALS

An early test of devil's claw in 1972 showed mild benefit in treating osteoarthrosis of the knee, but the herbal extract was injected directly into the affected joints.[47] In 1981, researchers saw no effect after giving 13 patients devil's claw extract for six weeks.[48] Other research, however, has generated positive results. Two uncontrolled European trials using 127 patients led to reductions in pain and better mobility; a Belgian study reported improvements rated "good" to "very good" in 60 of 84 patients.[49, 50]

Chinese doctors conducted three studies in 1994 and 1995 testing the effects of devil's claw in a total of 136 patients with osteoarthrosis, rheumatoid arthritis, or ankylosing spondylitis. All of the trials employed Pagosid, a proprietary extract of devil's claw that is widely available in the United States. According to the authors, clinical and laboratory measures of disease severity were both evaluated by standards set by the American College of Rheumatology.[51] The authors documented few side effects from Pagosid and no toxic changes to organs. Note: These studies were sponsored by the Swiss manufacturer of a proprietary devil's claw extract (Pagosid).

In the first study, each of 40 patients—20 with osteoarthrosis and 20 with rheumatoid arthritis—received 500 milligrams of Pagosid for four weeks. Doctors rated Pagosid effective in 85% of the osteoarthrosis patients, 90% of whom judged it effective. The authors reported improvement but no statistically significant changes in the rheumatoid arthritis patients—either because of the extremely short duration of study or a simple lack of efficacy.

In the second study, each of 38 patients with osteoarthrosis, rheumatoid arthritis, or ankylosing spondylitis received 1 gram of

Pagosid per day for four weeks. Doctors determined the drug to be effective in 85% of the osteoarthrosis patients, 75% of the rheumatoid arthritis patients, and 67% of the patients with ankylosing spondylitis.

In the third trial, rheumatologists studied the effects of Pagosid in 30 patients versus 28 controls who were given a common NSAID (diclofenac). Doctors rated Pagosid effective in 86.7% of the osteoarthrosis patients and 66.7% of the rheumatoid arthritis patients, with more of the osteoarthrosis patients enjoying excellent results. Overall, the controls taking diclofenac did not do as well (65% effective) as the thirty who took Pagosid (76.7% effective). One-quarter of the controls had to take medication to treat the gastric symptoms of diclofenac. A few of those receiving Pagosid had skin rashes that disappeared after the drug was discontinued.

NOTES

PREFACE: TAKE CHARGE OF YOUR HEALTH

1. *Am Pharm* 1990; NS30(7):10.

CHAPTER 1: OSTEOARTHROSIS (OSTEOARTHRITIS)

1. National Institute of Arthritis and Musculoskeletal and Skin Diseases.
2. Spector TD, et al. Genetic influences on osteoarthritis in women: A twin study. *Br Med J* 1996;312(7036):940–43.
3. Mapp PI, et al. Hypoxia, oxidative stress and rheumatoid arthritis. *Br Med Bull* 1995;51(2):419–36.
4. Spector TD, Hart DJ, Doyle DV. Incidence and progression of osteoarthritis in women with unilateral knee disease in the general population: the effect of obesity. *Ann Rheum Dis* 1994;53(9):565–68.

CHAPTER 2: PHYSICAL AND MENTAL THERAPIES

1. Ettinger W, et al. A randomized trial comparing aerobic exercise and resistance exercise with a health education program in older adults with osteoarthritis. The Fitness Arthritis and Seniors Trial. *JAMA* 1997;277(1):25–31.
2. *Tufts Diet Nutr Lett* 1996;14(5).

3. Daltroy LH, et al. Effectiveness of minimally supervised home aerobic training in patients with systemic rheumatic disease. *Br J Rheum* 1995;34:1064–69.
4. Greene, et al. Abstract presented at Clinical Research Meeting of the Association of American Physicians, American Society for Clinical Investigation, American Federation for Clinical Research. Baltimore, Maryland, April 30, 1994.
5. Takeda W, Wessel J. Acupuncture for the treatment of pain of osteoarthritic knees. *Arthritis Care Res* 1994;7(3):118–22.
6. Guan Z, Zhang J. Effects of acupuncture on immunoglobulins in patients with asthma and rheumatoid arthritis. *J Tradit Chin Med* 1995;15(2):102–5.
7. Ernst E . Acupuncture as a symptomatic treatment of osteoarthritis. A systematic review. *Scand J Rheumatol* 1997;26(6):444–47.
8. Liu X, et al. Effect of acupuncture and point-injection treatment on immunologic function in rheumatoid arthritis. *J Tradit Chin Med* 1993;13(3):174–78.

CHAPTER 3: ASPIRIN AND ITS OFFSPRING

1. Chrubasik S, et al. Evidence for antirheumatic effectiveness of *Herba Urtica dioicae* in acute arthritis: A pilot study. *Phytomedicine* 1997;4(2):105–8.
2. Ramm S, Hansen C. Brennesselblatter-extrakt bei arthrose und rheumatoider arthritis. *Therapiewoche* 1996;28:3–6 [In German].
3. Jack DB. One hundred years of aspirin. *Lancet* 1997;350(9075):437–39.
4. Dr. Sidney Wolfe, M.D., of Public Citizen Health Research Group, 1995 testimony at U.S. FDA hearing on NSAIDs.
5. Singh G et al. Gastrointestinal tract complications of nonsteroidal anti-inflammatory drug treatment in rheumatoid arthritis. A prospective observational cohort study. *Arch Intern Med* 1996;156(14):1530–36.
6. Hiroshowitz BI. NSAIDs and the gastrointestinal tract. *Gastroenterologist* 1994;2(3):207–23.
7. Brandt KD. Effects of NSAIDs on chondrocyte metabolism in vitro and in vivo. *Am J Med* 1987;83(5A):29–34.
8. Vidal y Plana RR, Karzel K. Glucosamine: Its importance for the metabolism of articular cartilage. II. Studies on articular cartilage *Fortschr Med* 1980;98(21):801–6 [In German].
9. Hunneyball IM. Some further effects of prednisolone and triamcinolone hexacetonide on experimental arthritis in rabbits. *Agents Actions* 1981;11(5):490–98.
10. Brooks PM, et al. NSAID and osteoarthritis: Help or hindrance? *J Rheumatol* 1982;9:3–5.
11. Bjarnason I, et al. Intestinal permeability and inflammation in rheumatoid arthritis: effects of non-steroidal anti-inflammatory drugs. *Lancet* 1984;2(8413):1171–74.
12. Hiroshowitz, 207-23.

13. Murphy PJ, Myers BL, Badia P. Nonsteroidal anti-inflammatory drugs alter body temperature and suppress melatonin in humans. *Physiol Behav* 1996;59:133–39.

14. Wolfe, 1995 FDA testimony.

15. Dr. Helen Shields, M.D., to *Boston Globe*, July 8, 1996.

16. Singh, 1530–36.

17. Akil M, et al. Infertility may sometimes be associated with NSAID consumption. *Br J Rheumatol* 1996;35:76–78.

18. Perneger TV, Whelton PK, and Klag MJ. Risk of kidney failure associated with the use of acetaminophen, aspirin, and nonsteroidal antiinflammatory drugs. *N Engl J Med* 1994;331(25):1675–79.

19. Singh, 1530–36.

20. Brandt, 29–34.

21. Newman NM and Ling RSM. Acetabular bond destruction related to nonsteroidal anti-inflammatory drugs. *The Lancet* 1985;2:11–13.

22. Singh, 1530–36.

23. Jack, 437–39.

24. Singh, 1530–36.

25. Hawkey CJ et al. Omeprazole compared with misoprostol for ulcers associated with nonsteroidal antiinflammatory drugs. Omeprazole versus Misoprostol for NSAID-induced Ulcer Management (OMNIUM) Study Group. *N Engl J Med* 1998;338(11):727–34.

26. Simon L, et al. Risk factors for serious nonsteroidal-induced gastrointestinal complications: Regression analysis of the MUCOSA trial. *Fam Medi* 1996; 28:204–10.

27. Brandt, 29–34.

28. Liu et al., 174–78.

29. Bjarnason, et al., 1117–74.

30. Hunneyball, 490–98.

31. Brooks et al., 3–5.

32. Newman and Ling, 11–13.

33. Dingle JT. The effect of NSAIDs on human articular cartilage glycosaminoglycan synthesis. *Eur J Rheumatol Inflamm* 1996;16:47–52.

34. Baggot JE, et al. Inhibition of folate dependent enzymes by NSAIDs. *Biochem J* 1992;282(Pt. 1):197–202.

35. Seibert K, et al. Mediation of inflammation by cyclooxygenase-2. *Agents Actions Suppl* 1995;46:41–50.

36. Strom BL. Adverse reactions to over-the-counter analgesics taken for therapeutic purposes. *JAMA* 1994;272(23):1866–67.

37. Perneger, Whelton, and Klag, 1675–79.

CHAPTER 4: THE CARTILAGE THERAPY REVOLUTION

1. Bland JH, Cooper SM. Osteoarthritis: Evidence for reversibility. *Semin Arthritis Rheum* 1984;14:106–33.
2. Perry GH, Smith MJG, Whiteside CG. Spontaneous recovery of the hip joint space in degenerative hip disease. *Ann Rheum Dis* 1972;31:440–48.
3. Setnikar I, et al. Pharmacokinetics of glucosamine in the dog and in man. *Arzneimmittelforschung* 1986;36:729–35 [In German].
4. Mankin HJ. Biochemical and metabolic aspects of osteoarthritis. *Orthop Clin North Am* 1972;2:19.
5. McCarty F. The neglect of gluscosamine as a treatment for osteoarthritis. *Medi Hypotheses* 1994;42(5):323–27.
6. Shield MJ. Anti-inflammatory drugs and their effects on cartilage synthesis and renal function. *Eur J Rheum Inflamm,* 1993;13:7–16.
7. Krajickova J, Macek J. Urinary proteoglycan degradation product excretion in patients with rheumatoid arthritis and osteoarthritis. *Ann Rheum Dis* 1988;47(6):468–71.
8. Setnikar I. Antireactive properties of chondroprotective drugs. *Int J Tissue React* 1992;14(5):253–61.
9. Vidal y Plana RR, Karzel K. Glucosamine: Its importance for the metabolism of articular cartilage. *Fortschr Med* 1980;98(21):801–6.
10. Prudden JF, et al. The discovery of a potent pure chemical wound healing accelerator. *Am Surg* 1970;19:560.
11. McCarty F. The neglect of gluscosamine as a treatment for osteoarthritis. *Med Hypotheses* 1994;42(5):323–27.
12. Setnikar, 253–61.
13. Lopez Vaz A. Double blind clinical evaluation of the relative efficacy of ibuprofen and glucosamine sulfate in the management of osteoarthrosis of the knee in out–patients. *Curr Med Res Opin* 1982;8(3):145–49.
14. Noack W, et al. Glucosamine sulfate in osteoarthritis of the knee. *Osteoarthritis Cartilage* 1994;2:51–59.
15. Reichelt A, et al. Efficacy and safety of intramuscular glucosamine sulfate in osteoarthritis of the knee. *Arzneimittelforschung* 1994;44(1):75–80 [In German].
16. D'Ambrosio E, et al. Glucosamine sulphate: A controlled clinical investigation in arthrosis. *Pharmatherapeutica* 1981;2(8):504–8 [In Italian].
17. Vajaradul Y. Double-blind clinical evaluation of intra-articular glucosamine in outpatients with gonarthritis. *Clin Ther* 1981;3(5):336–43.
18. Puljate JM, et al. Double blind clinical evaluation of oral glucosamine sulfate in the basic treatement of osteoarthrosis. *Curr Med Opin* 1980;7(2):110–14.
19. Rovati LC, et al. A large, randomized, placebo-controlled, double-blind study of glucosamine sulfate vs. piroxicam and vs. their association, on the kinetics of the symptomatic effect in knee osteoarthritis. *Osteoarthritis Cartilage* 1994;2(suppl. 1):56.

20. Crolle G, D'Este E. Glucosamine sulphate for the management of arthrosis: A controlled clinical investigation. *Curr Med Res Opin* 1980;7(2):104–9.

21. Muller-Fassbender H, et al. Glucosamine sulfate compared to ibuprofen in osteoarthritis of the knee. *Osteoarthritis Cartilage* 1994;2(1):61–69.

22. Dovanti A, Bignamini AA, Rovati AL. Therapeutic activity of oral glucosamine sulphate in osteoathrosis: A placebo-controlled double blind investigation. *Clin Ther* 1980;3(4):266–72.

23. Lopez, 145–49.

24. Noack et al., 51–59.

25. Reichelt et al., 75–80.

26. D'Ambrosio et al., 504–8.

27. Vajaradul, 336–43.

28. Puljate et al., 110–14.

29. Rovati et al., 56.

30. Sullivan MX, Hess WC. Cystine content of fingernails in arthritis. *J Bone Joint Surg* 1935;16:185–88.

31. Senturua BD. Results of treatment of chronic arthritis and rheumatoid conditions with colloidal sulfur. *J Bone Joint Surg* 1935;16:119–25.

32. Woldenburg SC. The treatment of arthritis with colloidal sulphur. *J South Med Assoc* 1935;28:875–81.

33. Karzel K, Domenjoz R. Effect of hexosamine derivatives and uronic acid derivatives on glycosaminoglycan metabolism of fibroblast cultures. *Pharmacology* 1971;5:337–45.

34. Caps JC, et al. Hexosamine metabolism. I. The absorption and metabolism in vivo of orally administered D-glucosamine and N-acetyl-glucosamine in the rat. *Biochem Biophys Acta* 1966;127:194–204.

35. Kohn P, et al. Metabolism of D-glucosamine and N-acetyl-glucosamine in the intact rat. *J Biol Chem* 1962;237(2):304–8.

36. Tesoriere G, et al. Intestinal absorption of glucosamine and N-acetyl-glucosamine. *Experientia* 1972;28:770–71.

37. Mazières B, et al. Chondroitin sulfate in the treatment of gonarthritis and coxarthritis: 5-months result of a multicenter double-blind controlled prospective study using placebo. *Rev Rhum Mal Osteoartic* 1992;59(7–8):466–72 [In French].

38. Rovetta G. Galactosaminogylcuronoglycan sulfate (matrix) in therapy of tibiofibular osteoarthritis of the knee. *Drugs Exp Clini Res* 1991;18(1):53–57.

39. Pipitone VR. Chondroprotection with chondroitin sulfate. *Drugs Exp Clini Res* 1991;17(1):3–7.

40. Oliviero U, et al. Effects of the treatment with matrix on elderly people with chronic articular degeneration. *Drugs Exp Clini Res* 1991;17(1):45–51.

41. Kerzberg EM, et al. Combination of glycosaminoglycans and acetylsalicylic acid in knee osteoarthrosis. *Scand J Rheumatol* 1987;16:377–80.

42. Mazières et al., 466–72.

43. Rovetta, 53–57.

44. Morrison M. Therapeutic applications of chondroitin sulfate: Appraisal of biologic properties. *Folia Angiol* 1977;25:225–32.

45. Soldani G. and Romagnoli J. Experimental and clinical pharmacology of glycosaminoglycans (GAGs). *Drugs Exp Clin Res* 1991;18(1):81–85.

46. Morrison, 225–32.

47. Soldani and Romagnoli, 81–85.

48. Baici A, et al. Analysis of glycosaminoglycans in human serum after oral administration of chondroitin sulfate. *Rheumatol Int* 1992;12(3):81–88.

49. Prudden JF, Balassa LL. The biological activity of bovine cartilage preparations. *Semin Arthritis Rheum* 1974;3(4):287–321.

50. Ibid.

51. Prudden JF. General Description of Catrix, Summary of Dosage Forms and The Results of Catrix Therapy. *The Journey,* a private publication of the Foundation for Cartilage and Immunology Research, 104 Post Office Road, Waccabuc, NY.

52. Rejholic V, et al. Long term studies of anti-osteoarthritic drugs. *Semin Arthritis Rheum* 1987;17(Suppl. 1):2.

53. Telephone conversation with J. F. Prudden, M.D., July 11, 1996.

54. Götz B. Well-nourished cartilage does not grind. *Arztk Praxus* 1982;34:3130–34 [In German].

55. Krug E. On supportive therapy for osteo- and chondropathies. *Z. Erfahrunsheilk* 1979;11:930–38 [In German].

56. Oberschelp U. Individual arthrosis therapy is possible. *Therapiewoche* 1985;44:5094–97 [In German].

57. Seeligmüller K, Happel KH. Can a mixture of gelatin and *L*-cystine stimulate proteoglycan synthesis? *Therapiewoche* 1989;39:3153–57 [In German].

58. Adam M. Osteoarthrosis therapy with gelatin preparations. *Therapiewoche* 1991;38:2456 [In German].

59. Ibid.

60. Reddy GK, et al. Urinary excretion of connective tissue metabolites under the influence of a new non-steroidal anti-inflammatory agent in adjuvant induced arthritis. *Agents Actions* 1987;22:99–105.

CHAPTER 5: GOUT

1. Bindoli A, et al. Inhibitory action of quercetin on xanthine oxidase and xanthine dehydrogenase activity. *Pharmacol Res Comm* 1985;17:831–39.

2. Lewis AS, et al. Inhibition of mammalian xanthine oxidase by folate compounds and amethopterin. *J Biol Chem* 1984;259:12–15.

3. Oster KA. Xanthine oxidase and folic acid. *Ann Intern Med* 1977;87:252.

4. Whitehead N, et al. Megaloblastic changes in the cervical epithelium: Association with oral contraceptive therapy and reversal with folic acid. *JAMA* 1973;226:1421–24.

5. Butterworth C, et al. Improvement in cervical dysplasia associated with folic acid therapy in users of oral contraceptives. *Am J Clin Nutr* 1982;35:73–82.

6. Blau LW. Cherry diet control for gout and arthritis. *Tex Rep Biol Med* 1950;8:309–11.

7. Kämpf R. *Schweiz Apotheker-Zeitung* 1976;114:337–42.

CHAPTER 6: RHEUMATIC DISEASES

1. National Institutes of Health; National Institute of Arthritis and Musculoskeletal and Skin Diseases. "Occurence and Impact of Rheumatoid Arthritis" (http://www.nih.gov/niam)

2. Jootsen LA, et al. Accelerated onset of collagen-induced arthritis by remote inflammation. *Clin Exp Immunol* 1994;97(2):204–11.

3. Mapp PI, et al. Hypoxia, oxidative stress and rheumatoid arthritis. *Br Med Bull* 1995;51(2):419–36.

4. Jaradaya A, et al. Erythrocyte antioxidant enzymes are reduced in patients with rheumatoid arthritis. *J Rheumatol* 1988;15(11):1628–31.

5. Harris ED. Pathogenesis of rheumatoid arthritis. *Am J Med* 1986;80(4B):4–10.

6. Chaitow L, Trenev N. *Probiotics.* Thorsons Publishers Ltd., Wellingborough, UK, 1990.

7. McDonagh JE, Walker DJ. Incidence of rheumatoid arthritis in a 10-year follow-up study of extended pedigree multicase families. *Br J Rheumatol* 1994;33(9):826–31.

8. Hall GM, Spector TD. Depressed levels of dehydroepiandrosterone sulphate in postmenopausal women with rheumatoid arthritis but no relation with axial bone density. *Ann Rheum Dis* 1993;52:211–14.

9. Sarzotti M, et al. Induction of protective CTL responses in newborn mice by a marine retrovirus. *Science* 1996;271(5256):1726–28.

10. Ridge JP, et al. Neonatal tolerance revisited: turning on newborn T cells with dendritic cells. *Science* 1996;271(5256):1723–26.

11. Forsthuber T, et al. Induction of TH1 and TH2 immunity in neonatal mice. *Science* 1996;271(5256):1728–30.

12. Sartor RB. Importance of intestinal mucosal immunity and luminal bacterial cell polymers in the aetiology of inflammatory joint diseases. *Baillieres Clin Rheumatol* 1989;3(2):223–45.

13. Trollmo C, et al. The gut as an inductive site for synovial and extra-articular immune responses in rheumatoid arthritis. *Ann Rheum Dis* 1994;53(6):377–82.

14. Weiner HL, et al. Oral tolerance: Immunologic mechanisms and treatment of animal and human organ-specific autoimmune diseases by oral adminstration of autoantigens. *Annu Rev Immunol* 1994;12:809–37.

15. Harris, 4–10.
16. Sydney B. Fibromyalgia and the rheumatisms. *Controv Rheumatol* 1993; 19(1):61–78.
17. Moldovsky HD, et al. Sleep, neuroimmune and neuroendocrine functions in fibromyalgia and chronic fatigue syndrome. *Adv Neuroimmunol* 995;5:39–56.
18. Wallace DJ, et al. Fibromyalgia, cytokines, fatigue syndromes and immune regulation. In: Friction JR, Awad E, eds. *Advances in Pain Research and Therapy,* vol. 17. New York: Raven Press, 1990:227–87.
19. Caruso I et al. Double-blind study of 5-hydroxytryptophan versus placebo in the treatment of primary fibromyalgia syndrome. *J Int Med Res* 1990;18(30):201–9.
20. Russell IJ et al. Treatment of fibromyalgia syndrome with Super Malic: a randomized, double blind, placebo controlled, crossover pilot study. *J Rheumatol* 1995;22(5):953–58.

CHAPTER 7:
GETTING THE RIGHT MEDICAL HELP

1. Hill J. An evaluation of the effectiveness, safety and acceptability of a nurse practitioner in a rheumatology outpatient clinic. *Br J Rheumatol* 1994;33(3):283–88.

CHAPTER 8: CONVENTIONAL MEDICINES
FOR RHEUMATIC DISEASES

1. *Fam Pract News* October 15, 1992.
2. Porter DL, et al. Outcome of secondary line therapy in rheumatoid arthritis. *Ann Rheum Dis* 1994;53(12):812–15.
3. Kushner. Does agressive therapy of rheumatoid arthritis affect outcomes? *J Rheumatol* 1989;16:1–4.
4. Wilkse KR, Healey L. Challenging the therapeutic pyramid: A new look at treatment strategies for rheumatoid arthritis. *J Rheumatol* 1990;17(Suppl. 25):4–7.
5. Epstein WV. Parenteral gold therapy for rheumatoid arthritis: A treatment whose time has gone. *J Rheumatol* 1989;16:1012:91–94.
6. Hill C et al. Neurological side effects in two patients receiving gold injections for rheumatoid arthritis. *Br J Rheumatol* 1995;34(10):989–90.
7. Harris ED. Hydrochloroquine is safe and probably useful in rheumatoid arthritis. *Ann Intern Med* 1993;119:1146–47.
8. De la Mata J, et al. Survival analysis of disease modifying antirheumatic drugs in Spanish rheumatoid arthritis patients. *Ann Rheum Dis* 1995;54(11):881–85.
9. Brennerman K, Suppressed Immune System Led to Death. *The News Tribune,* Framingham, MA, July 10, 1996.

10. Morgan SL. Supplementation with folic acid during methotrexate therapy for rheumatoid arthritis. A double-blind, placebo-controlled trial. *Ann Intern Med* 1994;121(11):833–41.

11. Segal R, et al. Methotrexate: Mechanism of action in rheumatoid arthritis. *Semin Arthritis Rheum* 1990;20(3):190–200.

12. De la Mata, et al., 881–85.

13. Tishler M, et al. Long-term experience with low dose MTX in rheumatoid arthritis. *Rheumatol Int* 1993;13(3):103–6.

14. Kremer J, et al. Study of use of methotrexate in the treatment of RA: Update after a mean of 90 months. *Arthritis Rheum* 1992;35(2):138–45.

15. Firestein GS. Mechanisms of methotrexate action in rheumatoid arthritis. *Arthritis Rheum* 1994; 37(2):193–200.

16. Alarcon GS, et al. Survival and drug discontinuation analyses in a large cohort of MTX treated rheumatoid arthritis patients. *Ann Rheum Dis* 1995; 54(9):708–12.

17. Tugwell P, et al. Combination therapy with cyclosporine and methotrexate in severe rheumatoid arthritis. *N Engl J Med* 1995;333:137–41.

18. Morgan, 833–41.

19. Weinblatt WE, et al. Long-term prospective trial of low dose methotrexate in rheumatoid arthritis. *Arthritis Rheum* 1988;31(2):167–75.

20. Morgan, 833–41.

21. Alarcon, 708–12.

CHAPTER 10: DIETARY THERAPY IN RHEUMATIC DISEASES

1. Esparza ML, Sasaki S, Kesteloot H. Nutrition, latitude, and multiple sclerosis: An ecological study. *Am J Epidemiol* 1995;142:733–37.

2. DeWitte TJ, et al. Hypochlorhydria and hypergastrinemia in rheumatoid arthritis. *Ann Rheum Dis* 1979;38:14–17.

3. Skoldstam L, Magnusson KE. Fasting, intestinal permeability and rheumatoid arthritis. *Rheum Dis Clin North Am* 1991;17(2):363–71.

4. Pamblad J, et al. Antirheumatic effects of fasting. *Rheum Dis Clin North Am* 1991;17(2):351–62.

5. Hafstrom I, et al. Effects of fasting on disease activity, neutrophil function, fatty acid composition and leukotriene biosynthesis in patients with rheumatoid arthritis. *Arthritis Rheum* 1988; 31(5):585–92.

6. Bricklin M. *The Practical Encyclopedia of Natural Healing* (New York: Penguin Books, 1983), 23. [Citing Lucas P and Power L, *JAMA*, April 9, 1982.]

7. Adam O. Low fat diet decreases alpha-tocopherol levels, and stimulates LDL oxidation and eicosanoid biosynthesis in man. *Eur J Med Res* 1995;1(2):65–71.

8. Munro R, Capell H. Prevalence of low body mass in rheumatoid arthritis: association with the acute phase response. *Ann Rheum Dis* 1997;56(5):326–29.

9. Kjeldsen-Kragh J, et al. Controlled trial of fasting and one year vegetarian diet in rheumatoid arthritis. *Lancet* 1991;338(8772):899–902.

10. Kjeldsen-Kragh J, et al. Changes in laboratory variables in rheumatoid arthritis patients during a trial of fasting and one-year vegetarian diet. *Scand J Rheumatol* 1995;24(2):85–93.

11. Darlington LG, et al. Placebo-controlled, blind study of dietary manipulation therapy in rheumatoid arthritis. *Lancet* 1986;1(8475):236–38.

12. Darlington LG; Ramsey NW. Review of dietary therapy for rheumatoid arthritis. *Br J Rheumatol* 1993;32(6):507–14.

13. Beri D, et al. Effect of dietary restrictions on disease activity in rheumatoid arthritis. *Ann Rheum Dis* 1988;47(1):69–72.

14. van de Laar MA, et al. Food intolerance in rheumatoid arthritis. II Clinical and histological aspects. *Ann Rheum Dis* 1991;51:303–6.

15. Haugen MA, et al. A pilot study of the effect of an elemental diet in the management of rheumatoid arthritis. *Clin Exp Rheumatol* 1994;12(3):235–39.

16. Panush RS, et al. Diet therapy for rheumatoid arthritis. *Arthritis Rheum* 1983;4:462–71.

17. Kjeldsen-Kragh J, et al. Antibodies against dietary antigens in rheumatoid arthritis patients treated with fasting and a one-year vegetarian diet. *Clin Exp Rheumatol* 1995;13:167–72.

18. Weiner HL, et al. Oral tolerance: Immunologic mechanisms and treatment of animal and human organ-specific autoimmune diseases by oral administration of autoantigens. *Annu Rev Immunol* 1994;12:809–37.

19. Sieper J, Mitchison AN. Therapy with oral type II collagen as a new possibility of selective immunosuppression in therapy of rheumatoid arthritis. *Z Rheumatol* 1994;53(2):53–58.

20. Trentham D, et al. Effects of oral administration of type II collagen on rheumatoid arthritis. *Science* 1993;261.

21. Rosenberg, Ronald. Autoimmune's Arthritis Drug Comes Up Short. *Boston Globe* May 13, 1997, page C-1.

22. Rosenberg, Ronald. Autoimmune Arthritis Drug Set For New Trials. *Boston Globe* May 6, 1998, page C-1.

CHAPTER 11: VITAMINS AND MINERALS

1. Kowsari B, et al. Assessment of the diet of patients with rheumatoid arthritis and osteoarthritis. *J Am Diet Assoc* 1983;82(6):657–59.

2. Kremer J, Bigdouette J. Nutrient intake of patients with rheumatoid arthritis is deficient in pyroxidine, zinc, copper, and magnesium. *J Rheumatol* 1996;23(6): 990–94.

3. Comstock GW, et al. Serum concentrations of alpha tocopherol, beta carotene, and retinol preceding the diagnosis of rheumatoid arthritis and systemic lupus erythematosus. *Ann Rheum Dis* 1997;56(5):323–25.

4. Kaufman W. The use of vitamin therapy to reverse certain concomitants of aging. *J Am Geriatr Soc* 1955;3:927.

5. Kaufman W. *The Common Form of Joint Dysfunction: Its Incidence and Treatment.* (Brattleboro, Vt: Hildreth, 1949).

6. Jonas WB, et al. The effect of niacinamide on osteoarthritis: A pilot study. *Inflamm Res* 1996;45:330–34.

7. Barton-Wright EC, Elliot WA. The pantothenic acid metabolism of rheumatoid arthritis. *Lancet* Oct. 26 1963:862.

8. Calcium pantothenate in arthritic conditions: A report from the General Practitioner Research Group. *Practitioner* 1980;224:208–11.

9. McAlindon TE, et al. Do antioxidant micronutrients protect against the development and progression of knee osteoarthritis? *Arthritis Rheum* 1996; 39(4):648–56.

10. Bates CJ. Proline and hydroxyline excretion and vitamin C status in elderly human subjects. *Clini Sci Mol Med* 1977;52:525–43.

11. Krystal G, et al. Stimulation of DNA synthesis by ascorbate in cultures of articular chondrocytes. *Arthritis Rheum* 1982;25:318–25.

12. Halliwell B, et al. *FEBS Lett* 1987;213(1):15–17.

13. Horrobin DF, et al. The regulation of prostaglandin E_1 formation: A candidate for one of the fundamental mechanisms involved in the actions of vitamin C. *Med Hypotheses* 1979;5(8):849–858.

14. Mitchell W. Allergies: Immediate-type hypersensitivity. *Protocol Botan Med* 1995;1(2):63–67. Herbal Research Publications, Ayer, MA.

15. Ibid.

16. McAlindon T, et al. Relation of dietary intake and serum levels of vitamin D to progression of osteoarthritis of the knee. *Ann Intern Med* 1996;125(5):353–59.

17. Kowsari et al., 657–59.

18. McAlindon, et al., 353–59.

19. Blankenhorn G. Clinical effectiveness of Spondyvit (vitamin E) in activated arthroses: A multicenter placebo-controlled double-blind study. *Z Orthop* 1986;124(3):340–43.

20. Edmonds SE, et al. Putative analgesic activity of repeated oral doses of vitamin E in the treatment of rheumatoid arthritis. *Ann Rheum Dis* 1997;56:649–55.

21. Schwartz ER. The modulation of osteoarthritic development by vitamins C and E. *Int J Vit Nutr Res* 1984;26:141–46.

22. Machtey I, et al. Tocopherol in osteoathritis: A controlled pilot study. *J Am Geriatr Soc* 1978;26:328–30.

23. Travers RL, et al. Boron and arthritis: the results of a double-blind pilot study. *J Nutr Med* 1990;1:127–32.

24. Newman RE. Arthritis or skeletal fluorosis and boron [Letter]. *Int Clin Nutr Rev* 1991;11(2):68–70; Newman RE. Boron beats arthritis. Proceedings of the ANZAAS Australian Academy of Science, Canberra, 1979.

25. Bruce A, et al. The effect of selenium and vitamin E on glutathione peroxidase levels and subjective symptoms in patients with arthrosis and rheumatoid arthritis. Proceedings of the New Zealand Workshop on Trace Elements in New Zealand. Dunedin University of Otago, 1981:92.

26. Ibid.

27. Jameson S, et al. Pain relief and selenium balance in patients with connective tissue disease and osteoarthritis: A double-blind selenium tocopherol study. *Nutr Res Suppl* 1985;(1):391–97.

28. Hill J, Bird HA. Failure of selenium-ACE to improve osteoarthritis. *Br J Rheumatol* 1990;29(3):211–13.

29. Simkin PA. Treatment of rheumatoid arthritis with oral zinc sulfate. Agents *Actions Suppl* 1981;8:8587–95.

30. Mattingly PC, Mowat AG. Zinc sulphate in rheumatoid arthritis. *Ann Rheum Dis* 1982;41:456–57.

31. Pandley SP, et al. Zinc in rheumatoid arthritis. *Indian J Med Res* 1985;81:618–20.

32. McAlindon, 648–56.

CHAPTER 12: TRADITIONAL HERBS

1. Weiner M. Ayurvedic medicinal plants. *Herbal HealthLine* 1991;2(2):1.

2. Opdyke DLJ. Fragrance raw materials monograph, olibanum gum. *Food Cosmet Toxicol* 1978;16:83.

3. Singh GB, Atal CK. Pharmacology of an extract of salai guggul ex-*Boswellia serrata*, a new non-steroidal anti-inflammatory agent. *Agents Actions* 1986;18(3/4):407–11.

4. Singh GB, et al. Abstract from the symposium on Recent Advances in Mediators of Inflammation and Anti-inflammatory Agents. Regional Research Laboratory, Jammu, India, 1984:38.

5. Singh GB, et al. Boswellic acids. *Drugs of the Future* 1993;19(4):307–9.

6. Gupta VN, et al. Pharmacology of the gum resin of *B. serrata*. *Indian Drugs* 1987;24(5):221–23.

7. Jiangsu Provincial Institute of Botany, 1990 Essentials of Medicinal Plants of New China, unpublished monograph.

8. Kiuchi F, et al. Inhibitors of prostaglandin biosynthesis from ginger. *Chem Pharm Bull (Tokyo)* 1982;30(2):754–57.

9. al-Yahya MA. Gastroprotective activity of ginger *Zingiber officinale rosc.*, in albino rats. *Am J Chin Med* 1989;17(1–2):51–56.

10. Kiuchi, et al., 754–57.

11. Suekawa M, et al. Pharmacological studies on ginger. IV. Effect of (6)-shogoal on the arachidonic cascade. *Nippon Yakurigaku Zasshi* 1986;88(4):263:9 [In Japanese].

12. *HerbalGram* 1993, No. 29:19, published by the American Botanical Council, Austin, Texas [citing *Folia Pharmacologica Japonica*, 1986;88(4):263–69.]

13. Kikuzaki H, Nakatani N. Antioxidant effects of some ginger constituents. *J Food Sci* 1993;58:1407.

14. Lee YB, et al. Antioxidant property in ginger rhizome and its application to meat products. *J Food Sci* 1986;51(1):20–23.

15. Saito Y, et al. The antioxidant effects of petroleum ether soluble and insoluble fractions from spices. *Eiyo To Shokuryo* 1976;29:505–10.

16. Kroes BH. Inhibition of human complement by beta-glycyrrhetinic acid, *Immunology* 1997; 90(1):115–20.

17. Oka H, et al. Prospective study of chemoprevention of hepatocellular carcinoma with Sho-saiko-to (TJ-9). *Cancer* 1995;76(5):743–49.

18. Ibid.

19. K Keller, R Hänsel, and RF Chandler, eds. *Adverse Effects of Herbal Drugs*, vol. 3. (Berlin, Heidelberg, New York: De Smet PAGM, Springer Verlag, 1997).

20. Lipsky PE, Tao XL. A potential new treatment for rheumatoid arthritis: thunder god vine. *Semin Arthritis Rheum* 1997;26(5):713–23.

21. Tao X. Effects of *Tripterygium wilfordii* hook F extracts on induction of cyclooxygenase 2 activity and prostaglandin E2 production. *Arthritis Rheum* 1998;41(1):130–38.; Tao X. The Chinese herbal remedy, T2, inhibits mitogen-induced cytokine gene transcription by T cells, but not initial signal transduction. *J Pharmacol Exp Ther* 1996;276(1):316–25.

22. *Tripterygium wilfordii* Research Group. Medical Information (Sanming District Second Hospital, Fujian). 1978;1–2:140.

23. Xu XY. *People's Mili Medi* 1980;3:38.

24. Kämpf, 337–42.

25. Lanhers MC, et al. Anti-inflammatory and analgesic effects of an aqueous extract of *Harpagophytum procumbens. Planta Med* 1992;58(2):117–23.

26. Blumenthal M et al. The Complete German Commission E Monographs: Therapeutic Guides to Herbal Medicines. Willow Bark, p. 230. American Botanical Council/Integrative Medicine Communications, Boston 1998.

27. Pattrick M, et al. Feverfew in rheumatoid arthritis: a double-blind placebo-controlled study. *Ann Rheum Dis* 1989;48(7):547–49.

28. Awang DV. *Can Pharm J* 1989;122(5):266.

29. Patrick, et al., 547–49.

30. Lewis DA, et al. *Int J Crude Drug Res* 1985;23(1):27.

31. Blumenthal M et al. The Complete German Commission E Monographs: Therapeutic Guides to Herbal Medicines. Celery, p. 320. American Botanical Council/Integrative Medicine Communications, Boston 1998.

32. Bingham R, et al. Yucca plant saponin in the management of arthritis. *J Appl Nutr* 1975;27:45–50.

33. Morales, et al. The effect of lipopolysaccharides on the biosynthesis and release of proteoglycans from calf articular cartilage cultures. *J Biol Chem* 1984;259:6720–29.

CHAPTER 13: NUTRACEUTICAL REMEDIES FROM NATURE

1. Haugen MA, et al. Changes in plasma phospholipid fatty acids and their relationship to disease activity in rheumatoid arthritis patients treated with a vegetarian diet. *Br J Nutr* 1994;72(4):555–66.

2. Fortin PR, et al. Validation of a meta-analysis: The effects of fish oil in rheumatoid arthritis. *J Clin Epidemiol* 1995;48(11):1379–90.

3. Geusens P, et al. Long term effect of omega-3 fatty acid supplementation in active rheumatoid arthritis: A 12-month, double-blind controlled study. *Arthritis Rheum* 1994;37(6):824–29.

4. Kremer JM, et al. Effects of high dose fish oil on rheumatoid arthritis after stopping NSAIDs: Clinical and immune correlates. *Arth Rheum* 1995; 38(8):1107–14.

5. Bittiner S, et al. A double-blind, randomized, placebo-controlled trial of fish oil in psoriasis. *Lancet,* Feb. 20 1988;1:378–80.

6. Shukla VKS, et al. The presence of oxidative polymeric materials in encapsulated fish oils. *Lipids* 1988;26:23–26.

7. Shapiro et al. Diet and rheumatoid arthritis in women: A possible protective effect of fish consumption. *Epidemiology* 1996;7:256–63.

8. Nordstrom DC, et al. Alpha-linolenic acid in the treatment of rheumatoid arthritis. A double-blind, placebo-controlled and randomized study: flaxseed vs. safflower seed. *Rheumatol Int* 1995;14(6):231–34.

9. Mantizioni E, et al. Dietary substitution with alpha-linolenic acid-rich vegetable oil increases eicosapentaenoic acid concentrations in tissues. *Am J Clin Nutr* 1994;59:1304–309.

10. Leventhal L, et al. Treatment of rheumatoid arthritis with GLA. *Ann Intern Med* 1993;119:867–73.

11. Brzeski M, et al. Preliminary report: EPO in patients with rheumatoid arthritis and side-effects of NSAIDs. *Br J Rheumatol* 1991;30:370.

12. Watson J, et al. Cytokine and prostaglandin production by monocytes of volunteers and rheumatoid arthritis patients treated with dietary supplements of black currant seed oil. *Br J Rheumatol* 1993;32(12):1055–58.

13. Zurier RB, et al. Gamma-linolenic treatment of rheumatoid arthritis: A randomized, placebo-controlled trial. *Arthritis Rheum* 1996;39(11):1808–17.

14. Rothman D, DeLuca P, Zurier RB. Botanical lipids: effects on inflammation, immune responses, and rheumatoid arthritis. *Semin Arthritis Rheum* 1995;25(2):87–96.

15. Byars ML, Watson J, McGill PE. Black currant seed oil as a source of polyunsaturated fatty acids in the treatment of inflammatory disease. *Biochem Soc Trans* 1992;20(2):139S.

16. Jäntti J, et al. EPO in rheumatoid arthritis: Changes in serum lipids and fatty acids. *Ann Rheum Dis* 1989;48:124–27.

17. Siemandi H. The effect of *cis*-9-cetyl myristoleate (CMO) and adjunctive therapy on arthritis and auto-immune disease: A randomized trial. *Townsend Letter for Doctors*, August 1997, 58–63.

18. Prudden JF and Balassa LL. The biological activity of bovine cartilage preparations. *Semin Arthritis Rheum* 1974;3(4):287–321.

19. Moses MA. A cartilage-derived inhibitor of neovascularization and metalloproteinases. *Clin Exp Rheumatol* 1993;8(suppl. 11):S67–S69.

20. Kuettner K, Pauli B. Inhibition of neovascularization by a cartilage factor. *Ciba Found Symp* 1983;100:163–73.

21. Colville-Nash PR, Scott DL. Angiogenesis and rheumatoid arthritis: Pathogenic and therapeutic implications. *Ann Rheum Dis* 1992;51(7):919–25.

22. Kamel M, Alnahdi M. Inhibition of superoxide anion release from human polymorphonuclear leukocytes by N-acetyl-galactosamine and N-acetyl-glucosamine. *Clin Rheumatol* 1992;11:254–60.

23. Prudden and Balassa, 287–321.

24. Byars ML, et al., 1395.

25. Telephone conversation with Dr. John F. Prudden, July 11, 1996.

26. Prudden and Balassa, 287–321.

27. Deal CL, et al. Treatment of arthritis with topical capsaicin: A double-blind trial. *Clin Ther* 1991;13(3):383–95; McCarthy GM, McCarty DJ. Effect of topical capsaicin in the therapy of painful osteoarthritis of the hands. *J Rheumatol* 1992;19(4):604–07.

28. Rao CV, et al. Antioxidant activity of curcumin and related compounds: Lipid peroxide formation in experimental inflammation. *Cancer Res* 1993;55:259.

29. Sharma SC, et al. Lipid peroxide formation in experimental inflammation. *Biochem Pharmacol* 1972;21:1210.

30. Soni KB, Kuttan R. Effect of oral curcumin administration on serum peroxides and cholesterol levels in human volunteers. *Indian J Physiol Pharmacol* 1992;36(4):273–75.

31. Srinivas L, Shalini VK, Shylaja M. Turmerin: a water soluble antioxidant peptide from turmeric. *Arch Biochem Biophys* 1992;292(2):617–23.

32. Srivasta R, Srimal RC. Modification of certain inflammation-induced biochemical changes by curcumin. *Indian J Med Res* 1985;81:215–23.

NOTES

33. Srimal R, Dhawan B. Pharmacology of diferuloyl methane (curcumin), a non-steroidal anti-inflammatory agent. *J Pharm Pharmacol* 1973;25(6):447–52.
34. Deodhar SD, et al. Preliminary studies on antirheumatic activity of curcumin (diferuloyl methane). *Indian J Med Res* 1980;71:632.
35. Satsokar RR, et al. Evaluation of antiinflammatory property of curcumin in patients with post-operative inflammation. *Int J Clin Pharmacol Toxicol* 1986; 24:651.
36. Schwitters, Bert and Jacques Masquelier. *OPC in Practice* (Rome, Italy: Alfa Omega Editrice, 1993), 112. [Citing Dubos G, et al. *Rev Geriatr* 1980; 5(6); Beylot C, et al. *Gaz Med France* 1980;87(22).]
37. Ibid., 58. [Citing Pfister A, Simon MT, Gazave JM. Fixation sites of procyanidolic oligomers in the blood capillary walls of the lungs of guinea pigs. *Acta Ther* 1982;8.]
38. Ibid., 148 [Citing Masquelier J, et al. *Acta Ther* 1981;7:101–105.]
39. Ibid. [Citing Tixier JM, et al. Evidence by in vivo and in vitro studies that binding of pycnogenols to elastin affects its rate of degradation by elastases. *Biochem Pharmacol* 1984;33(24):3933–39; Tixier, JM, et al. Biochemistry and Connective Tissue Laboratory, University of Paris, June 25, 1984.]
40. Kuttan R, et al. Collagen treated with (+) catechin becomes resistant to the action of mammalian collagenases. *Experientia* 1981;37(3):221–23.
41. Tixier, et al., 3933–39.
42. Kakegawa, et al. Inhibitory effects of tannins on hyaluronidase activation and on the degranulation from rat mesentry mast cells. *Chem Pharm Bull (Tokyo)* 1985;33(11):3079–82.
43. Schwitters and Masquelier, 129. [Citing Mori, et al. *Med Sci Res* 1987;15: 831–32.]
44. U.S. patent no. 4,698, 360. Oct 6, 1987.
45. Laparra J, et al. Original work. University of Bordeaux, 1976.
46. Gabor M, et al. Effects of benzopyrone derivatives on simultaneously induced croton oil ear oedema and carrageenen [sic] paw oedema in rats. *Acta Physiol Hung* 1991;77(3–4):197–207.
47. Parienti J, et al. Means of controlling post traumatic edema in sports injuries with l'Endotélon [OPC]. *Gaz Med France* 1983;90(3).
48. Masquelier, Jacques. Pycnogenols: Recent Advances in the Therapeutical Activity of Procyanidins. *Natural Products as Medicinal Agents* (Stuttgart: Hyppocrates Verlag, 1981).
49. Blaszo G, Gabor M. Edema-inhibiting effect of procyanidin. *Acta Physiol Acad Hung* 1985;65(2):235–40.
50. Kakegawa, et al., 3079–82.
51. Bombardelli E, et al. Botanical derivatives in functional cosmetics. *Drug Cosmet Ind* 1994;155:44–51.
52. Telephone conversation with John F. Prudden, M.D., July 11, 1996.

53. Felton GE. *Hawaii Med J* 1977;36(2):39.

54. Steffen C, Menzel J. Basic studies on enzyme therapy of immune complex diseases. *Wien Klin Wochenschr* (Vienna Clinical Weekly) 1985;97(8):376–385 [In German].

55. Miehle W. Controversial and so-called alternative therapeutic approaches. *Z Rheumatol* 1987;46(1):1–12 [In German].

56. Cichoke AJ. Treating rheumatoid arthritis with enzymes. *Townsend Letter for Doctors and Patients* January 1996; pp. 32–34. [Citing Uffelmann K, et al. *Allgemain Med* 1990;19:151–53 (In German).]

57. Ibid. 32–34. [Citing Vogler W. *Naturund GanzheitsMed* 1988;1:123–25 (In German).]

58. Ibid. 32–34. [Citing Eberle R. *Therapiewoche* 1987;37:7 (In German).]

59. Ibid. [Citing Horger I, et al. *Naturund GanzheitsMed* 1988;1:117–22 (In German).]

60. Steffen C, et al. Enzyme therapy in comparison with immune complex determinations in chronic polyarthritis. *Z Rheumatol* 1985;44(2):51–56. [In German]; Steffen C, Menzel J. Basic studies on enzyme therapy of immune complex diseases. *Wien Klin Wochenschr (Vienna Clinical Weekly)* 1985;97(8):376–85. [In German.]

61. Cichoke, 32–34. [Citing Klein G, et al. *Allgemein Med* 1990;144–47 (In German).]

62. Ibid. [Citing Klein G, et al. *Naturund GanzheitsMed* 1988;1:112–16 (In German).]

63. Ibid. [Citing Gallachi G. *Allgemein Med* 1990 19:148–50 (In German).]

64. Bombardelli et al., 44–51.

65. Felton, 39.

66. Taussig S. The mechanism of the physiological action of bromelain. *Med Hypothesis* 1980;6:99–104.

67. Cohen A, Goldman J. Bromelains therapy in rheumatoid arthritis. *Penn Med J* 1964;67:27–30.

68. Netti C, Bandi GL, Pecile A. Anti-inflammatory action of proteolytic enzymes of animal vegetable or bacterial origin administered orally compared with that of known anti-phlogistic compounds. *Farmaco [Prat]* 1972;27(8):453–66.

69. Hazelton RA. Rheumatology Department, University of Queensland Medical Center, Queensland, Australia. As summarized by Walker M, *Townsend Letter for Doctors*, October 1990.

70. Gibson RG, et al. Green lipped mussel extract in arthritis. [Letter.] *Lancet*, 1981;1(8217):439.

71. Gibson RG, et al. *Perna canaliculus* in the treatment of arthritis. *Practitioner* 1980;224:955–60.

CHAPTER 14: ANTIBIOTIC THERAPY

1. Trentham DE, Dynesius-Trentham RA. Antibiotic therapy for rheumatoid arthritis. Scientific and anecdotal appraisals. *Rheum Dis Clin North Am* 1995;21(3):817–34.

2. Wilder RW. Rheumatoid arthritis: Etiology. In: *Primer on Rheumatic Diseases,* 10th ed., (Atlanta: Arthritis Foundation, 1993).

3. Webster ADB, et al. Critical dependence on antibody for defense against mycoplasmas. *Clin Exp Immunol* 1988;71:383–87.

4. Cole BC, et al. Mycoplasma-induced arthritis. In: *The Mycoplasmas,* vol. 4. (New York: Academic Press, 1985), 107.

5. Khare SD, Luthra HS, David CS. Spontaneous inflammatory arthritis in HLA-B27 transgenic mice lacking beta 2-microglobulin: a model of human spondyloarthropathies. *J Exp Med* 1995;182(4):1153–58.

6. Seitz M, et al. Enhanced interferon-gamma production by lymphocytes induced by a mitogen from mycoplasma in patients with ankylosing spondylitis. *Rheumatol Int* 1989;9(2):85–90.

7. Webster et al., 383–87.

8. Furr PM, et al. Mycoplasmas and ureaplasmas in patients with hypogammaglobulinaemia and their role in arthritis: Microbiological observations over twenty years. *Ann Rheum Dis* 1994;53:183–87.

9. Webster et al., 383–87.

10. Ibid.

11. So AKL, et al. Arthritis caused by *Mycoplasma salivarium* in hypogammaglobulinaemia. *Br J Rheumatol* 1983;286:762–63.

12. Furr et al., 183–87.

13. Webster et al., 383–87.

14. Furr et al., 183–87.

15. Tumiati B, et al. High dose immunoglobin therapy as an immunomodulatory treatment of rheumatoid arthritis. *Arthritis Rheum* 1992;35:10,1126–33.

16. Gelfand EW. Unique susceptibility of patients with antibody deficiency to mycoplasma infection. *Clin Infect Dis* 1993;17(suppl.):S250–53.

17. Sabin AB, et al. Search for micoorganisms of the pleuro pneumoniae group in rheumatic and nonrheumatic children. *Proc Soc Exp Biol Med* 1940;44:569–71.

18. Swift HF, Brown TMcP. Pathogenic pleuro pneumonia-like micoorganisms from acute rheumatic exudates and tissues. *Science* 1939;89 (2308):271–72.

19. McPherson-Brown T, et al. Antibiotic therapy of rheumatoid arthritis: A retrospective cohort study of 98 patients with 451 patient-years of follow-up. *Congress of Rheumatology* 1985:S85.

20. Ibid.

21. Levinski WK, Lansbury J. An attempt to transmit rheumatoid arthritis to humans. *Proc Soc Exp Biol Med* 1951;78.

22. Skinner M, et al. Tetracycline in the treatment of rheumatoid arthritis: A doubler blind controlled study. *Arthritis Rheum* 1971; 14:727–32.

23. Scammell H. *The Arthritis Breakthrough* (New York: M. Evans and Company, 1993), 37. [Citing the *Wall Street Journal,* June 5, 1987.]

24. Sanchez L. Tetracyline treatment in rheumatoid arthritis and other rheumatic diseases. *Braz J Med* 1968;82:21–31.

25. Cantwell AR, et al. Acid-fast bacteria as a possible cause of scleroderma. *Dermatologica* 1968;136:141–50.

26. Ennis RS, et al. Persistent *Mycoplasma hyorhinis* (MH) antigen in chronic mycoplasmal arthritis of swine. *Arthritis Rheum* 1972;15:108.

27. Smith DE, et al. Experimental bedsonial arthritis. *Arthritis Rheum* 1973;16:21–29.

28. Jansson E, et al. Mycoplasmas and arthritis. *Z Rheumatol* 1983;42(6):315–19.

29. Taylor-Robinson D. Mycoplasmal arthritis in man. *Isr J Med Sci* 1981; 17(7):616–21.

30. Gorina LG, et al. Laboratory diagnosis of human *Mycoplasma* infection. *Vestn Akad Med Nauk SSSR* 1991;6:44–47 [In Russian].

31. Clark HW, et al. Detection of mycoplasmal antigens in immune complexes from rheumatoid arthritis synovial fluids. *Ann Allergy* 1988;60(5):394–98.

32. Gorina LG, et al. Detection of mycoplasmal arthritidis and *M. fermentans* antibodies in rheumatoid arthritis patients by an immunoenzyme method. *Zh Mikrobiol Epidemiol Immunobiol* 1985;6:48–52 [In Russian].

33. Zheverzheeva IV, et al. Indication of mycoplasmas in the synovial fluid of rheumatoid arthritis patients. *Zh Mikrobiol Epidemiol Immunobiol* 1983;9:63–69 [In Russian].

34. Jansson E, et al. Cultivation of fastidious mycoplasmas from human arthritis. *Z Rheumatol* 1983;42(2):66–69.

35. Taylor-Robinson D, et al. Detection of *Chlamydia thachomatis* DNA in joints of reactive arthritis patients by polymerase chain reaction. *The Lancet* 1992;340:81–82.

36. Ginsburg KS, et al. *Urealyplasma urealyticum* and *Mycoplasma hominis* in women with systemic lupus erythematosus. *Arthritis Rheum* 1992;35(4):429–43.

37. Cantwell AR, et al. Acid-fast bacteria in scleroderma and morphea. *Arch Dermatol* 1971;104:21–25.

38. Cantwell AR, et al. Histologic observations of coccoid forms suggestive of cell wall deficient bacteria in cutaneous and systemic SLE. *Int J Dermatol* 1982;21(9):526–37.

39. Ginsburg et al., 429–43.

40. Brown T, et al. Antimycoplasma approach to the mechanism and the control of rheumatoid disease. In: *Inflammatory Diseases and Copper* (Totowa, N.J.: Humana Press, 1982).

41. Gelfand EW, S250–53.

42. The Arthritis Foundation. *Understanding Arthritis,* Irving Kushner, Ann Forer, and Ann McGuire, eds. New York: Charles Scribner's Sons/Macmillan, 1984.

43. Clark HW, et al. Detection of mycoplasmal antigens in immune complexes from rheumatoid arthritis synovial fluids. *Ann Allergy* 1988;60(5):394–98.

44. Gorina LG, et al. Mycoplasmal arthritis in man and mechanisms of its pathogenesis. *Vestn Akad Med Nauk SSSR* 1989;6:84–87 [In Russian].

45. Sakkas LI, et al. Interleukin-12 is expressed by infiltrating macrophages and synovial lining cells in rheumatoid arthritis and osteoarthritis. *Cell Immunol* 1998;188(2):105–10; Qin S, et al. The chemokine receptors CXCR3 and CCR5 mark subsets of T cells associated with certain inflammatory reactions. *J Clin Invest* 1998;101(4):746–54; Kroemer G, et al. Differential involvement of Th1 and Th2 cytokines in autoimmune diseases. *Autoimmunity* 1996;24(1):25–33 [Review].

46. McPherson-Brown, et al., S85.

47. Gelfand EW. Unique susceptibility of patients with antibody deficiency to mycoplasma infection. *Clin Infect Dis* 1993;17(suppl):S250–53.

48. Kloppenburg M, et al. Minocycline in active rheumatoid arthritis: A double-blind placebo-controlled trial. *Arthritis Rheum* 1994;37:629–36.

49. Langevitz P, et al. Treatment of resistant rheumatoid arthritis with minocycline: An open study. *J Rheumatol* 1992;19:1502–04.

50. Breedveld FC, et al. Minocycline treatment for rheumatoid arthritis: An open dose finding study. *J Rheumatol* 1990;17:43–46.

51. Paulus HE. Minocyline treatment of rheumatoid arthritis. *Ann Intern Med* 1995;122:147–48.

52. Tilley B, et al. Minocycline in rheumatoid arthritis: A 48-week, double-blind, placebo-controlled study. *Ann Intern Med* 1995;122:81–89.

53. Raymond Gordon, Ph.D. Emeritus at Antioch College. Letter to *The Intercessor,* The Road Back Foundation, 4985 North Lake Hill Road, Delaware, OH, Nov. 1995.

54. O'Dell JR, et al. Treatment of early rheumatoid arthritis with minocycline or placebo: Results of a randomized, double-blind, placebo-controlled trial [Comments]. *Arthritis Rheum* 1997;40(5):794–96, 842–48.

55. Nip LH, et al. Inhibition of epethelial cell matrix metalloproteinases by tetracyclines. *J Periodont Res* 1993;28:379–85.

56. Sorsa T, et al. Collagenase in synovitis of rheumatoid arthritis. *Semin Arthritis Rheum* 1992;22:44–53.

57. Golub LM, et al. Host modulation with tetracyclines and their chemically modified analogues. *Curr Opin Dent* 1992;2:80–90.

58. Ibid.

59. Pruzanski W, et al. Inhibition of enzymatic activity of phospholipases A2 by minocycline and doxycycline. *Biochem Pharmacol* 1992;44:1165–70.

60. Kloppenburg M, et al. Minocycline inhibits T cell proliferation and interferon gamma (IFN-gamma) production after stimulation with anti-CD3 monoclonal antibodies *Br J Rheumatol* 1992;31:S41.

CHAPTER 15: HOMEOPATHIC REMEDIES

1. Gibson RG. Homoeopathic therapy in rheumatoid arthritis: evaluation by double-blind clinical therapeutic trial. *Br J Clin Pharmacol* 1980;9(5):453–59.
2. Shipley M. Controlled trial of homoeopathic treatment of osteoarthritis. *Lancet* 1983;1(8316):97–98.

CHAPTER 16: FOLK REMEDIES

1. Malanow MR, et al. Systemic lupus erythematosus–like syndrome in monkeys fed alfalfa sprouts: Role of a non-protein amino acid. *Science* 1982;216:415–17.
2. Roberts JL, Hayashi JA. Exacerbation of SLE associated with alfalfa ingestion [Letter]. *N Engl J Med* 1983;308(22):1361.

APPENDIX C: TOP HERBS–SCIENTIFIC SUMMARIES

1. Singh GB, Atal CK. Pharmacology of an extract of salai guggul ex-*Boswellia serrata*, a new non-steroidal anti-inflammatory agent. *Agents Actions* 1986;18(3/4):407–11.
2. Annual Report. Regional Research Laboratory, Jammu, India, 1987–1988:1–2.
3. Duwiejua M, et al. Anti-inflammatory activity of resins from some species of the plant family *Burseraceae*. *Planta Med* 1993;59(1):12–16.
4. Safayi H, et al. Boswellic acids: Novel, specific, non-redox inhibitors of 5-lipoxygenase. *J Pharmacol Exp Ther* 1992;261(3):1143.
5. Singh, Atal, 407–11.
6. Sharma ML, et al. Effect of saai guggal, ex-*Boswellia serrata*, on cellular and humoral immune response and leucocyte migration. *Agents Actions* 1988; 24:161–64.
7. Sharma ML, et al. Anti-arthritic activity of boswellic acids in bovine serum albumin-induced arthritis. *Int J Immunopharmacol* 1989;11(6):647–52.
8. Kapil A, Moza N. Anti-complementary activity of boswellic acids—an inhibitor of C-3 convertase of the classical complement pathway. *Int J Immunopharmacol* 1992;14(7):1139–43.
9. Singh GB, et al. Abstract from the symposium on Recent Advances in Mediators of Inflammation and Anti-inflammatory Agents. Regional Research Laboratory, Jammu, India, 1984:38.
10. Reddy GK, et al. Urinary excretion of connective tissue metabolites under the influence of a new non-steroidal anti-inflammatory agent in adjuvant induced arthritis. *Agents Actions* 1987;22:99–105.
11. Gupta VN, et al. Pharmacology of the gum resin of *B. serrata*. *Indian Drugs* 1987;24(5):221–23.

12. Majeed M, et al. "Boswellin, the Anti-Inflammatory Phytonutrient," p. 50. Nutriscience Publishers, Inc. Piscataway, New Jersey. [Citing Pachnanda VK, et al. *Ind J Pharm* 1981;(13):63.]

13. Annual Report. Regional Research Laboratory, Jammu, India, 1987–1988: 1–2.

14. Singh GB, et al. New phytotherapeutic agent for treatment of arthritis and allied disorders with novel mode of action. Presented at the Fourth Annual International Congress on Phytotherapy, September 1992, Munich, Germany, [Abstract SL 74].

15. Annual Report, Regional Research Laboratory, Jammu, India, 1987–1988: 1–2.

16. Srivastava KC, Mustafa T. Ginger (*Zingiber offincinale*) and rheumatic disorders. *Med Hypotheses* 1989;29(1):25–28.

17. Srivastava KC, Mustafa T. Ginger (*Zingiber offincinale*) in rheumatic and musculoskeletal disorders. *Med Hypotheses* 1992;39(4):342–48.

18. Cyong JA. A pharmacological study of the anti-inflammatory activity of Chinese herbs: A review. *Int J Acupunct Electrother Res* 1982;7(2–3):173–202.

19. Hashimoto, et al. Effects of saikosaponins on liver tyrosine aminotransfer activity induced by cortisone in adrenalectomized rats. *Planta Med* 1985;5:401–3.

20. Ohuchi K, et al. Pharmacological influence of saikosaponins on prostaglandin E2 production by peritoneal macrophages. *Planta Med* 1985 June;(3):208–12.

21. Yamammoto M, et al. Structure and action of saikosaponins isolated from *Bupleurum falcatum* L. *Arzneimittelforschung* 1975;25:1021–40.

22. Zhongchu A, et al. The anti-allergic inflammation action of saikosaponins. *J Tradit Chin Med* 1983;3(2):103–12.

23. Bermejo Benito P, et al. In vivo and in vitro antiinflammatory activity of saikosaponins. *Life Sci* 1998;63(13):1147–56; Cyong JC. [New BRM from kampoherbal medicine]. *Nippon Yakurigaku Zasshi* 1997;110 Suppl 1:87P–92P [In Japanese]; Kanauchi H, et al. Evaluation of the Japanese-Chinese herbal medicine, kampo, for the treatment of lupus dermatoses in autoimmune prone MRL/Mp-lpr/lpr mice. *J Dermatol* 1994;21(12):935–39.

24. Matsumoto T, et al. Effect of licorice roots on carageenan-induced decrease in immune complexes clearance in mice. *J Ethnopharmacol* 1996;53:1–4.

25. Amagaya S, Ogihara Y. Effects of Shosaikoto on plasma catecholamines. *J Ethnopharmacol* 1989;26(3):271–76.

26. Hashimoto, et al., 401–3.

27. Amagaya S, et al. Effects of Shosaikoto, an Oriental herbal medicinal mixture, on restraint-stressed mice. *J Ethnopharmacol* 1990;28:357–63.

28. Iwama H, et al. Studies of the combined use of steroid and Shosaikoto, one of the Kampohozai (TCM), on pituitary adrenocortical axis function and immune responses. *J Pharmacobiodyn* 1986;9(2):189–96.

29. Nagatsu Y, et al. Modification of macrophage functions by Shosaikoto (kampo medicine) leads to enhancement of immune response. *Chem Pharm Bull (Tokyo)* 1989;37(6):1540–42.

30. Amagaya et al., 357.

31. Ye WH. Mechanism of treating rheumatoid arthritis with polyglycosides of *Tripterygium wilfordii* Hook (T II). III. Study on inhibitory effect of T II on in vitro Ig secreted by peripheral blood mononuclear cells from normal controls and RA patients. *Chung Kuo I Hsueh Ko Hsueh Yuan Hsueh Pao* 1990;12(3):217–22 [In Chinese].

32. Yao Q, Zgang N. Effects of tripclorlide (T4) of *Tripterygium wilfordii* Hook on peripheral blood mononuclear cells of rheumatoid arthritis patients. *Chung Kuo I Hsueh Yuan Hseuh Pao* 1994;(5):352–55.

33. Yu KT, et al. Inhibition of IL-1 release from human monocytes and suppression of streptoccal cell wall and adjuvant-induced arthritis in rats by an extract of *Tripterygium wilfordii* Hook. *Gen Pharmacol* 1994;25(6):1115–22.

34. Gu WZ, et al. Inhibition of type II collagen-induced arthritis in mice by an immunosuppressive extract of *Tripterygium wilfordii* Hook f. *J Rheumatol* 1992;19(5):682–88.

35. Tao X, et al. Effect of an extract of the Chinese herbal remedy *Tripterygium wilfordii* Hook F on human immune responsiveness. *Arthritis Rheum* 1991;34(10):1274–81.

36. Tao XL. Mechanism of treating rheumatoid arthritis with *Tripterygium wilfordii* hook. II. Effect on PGE$_2$ secretion *Chung Kuo I Hsueh Yuan Hseuh Pao* 1989;11(1):36–40 [In Chinese].

37. Zhang MM, et al. Effect of *Tripterygium wilfordii* on adrenal cortex in rat with adjuvant arthritis. *J Tongi Med Univ* 1994;14(3):158–61.

38. Deyong Y. Clinical observation of 144 cases of rheumatoid arthritis treated with glycoside of radix *Tripterygium wilfordii*. *J Tradit Chin Med* 1983;3(2):125–29.

39. Ibid.

40. Tao XL. A prospective, controlled double-blind cross-over study of *Tripterygium wilfordii* Hook F in treatment of rheumatoid arthritis. *Chin Med J (Engl)* 1989;102(5):327–32.

41. Tao X, Sun Y, Zhang N. Treatment of RA with low doses of multi-glycosides of *Tripterygium wilfordii*. *Chung Msi I Chieh Ho Tsa Chih* 1990;102(5):327–32 [In Chinese].

42. Wanzhang Q, et al. Clinical observations on *Tripterygium wilfordii* in treatment of 26 cases of discoid erythematosus: Report of 103 cases. *Chin Med J (Engl)* 1983;3(2):131–32.

43. Wanzhang Q, et al. *Tripterygium wilfordii* hook F. in systemic lupus erythematosus: Report of 103 cases. *Chin Med J (Engl)* 1981;94:827–34.

44. Erdos A. Contribution to the pharmacology and toxicology of different extracts as well as the harpagosid from *Harpagophytum procumbens* DC. *Planta Med* 1978;34(1):97–108 [In German].

45. McLeod DW, Revell P, Robinson BV. Investigations of *Harpagophytum procumbens* (Devil's Claw) in the treatment of experimental inflammation and arthritis in

NOTES

the rat. *Br J Pharmacol* 1979;66(1):140P–41P; Eichler O, Koch C. Antiphlogistic, analgesic and spasmolytic effect of harpagoside, a glycoside from the root of *Harpagophytum procumbens* DC. *Arzneimittelforschung* 1970; 20(1):107–9 [In German].

46. Lahners, et al., 117.
47. Schmidt S. *Therapiewoche* 1972;13:1072.
48. Grahame R, Robinson BV. Devil's Claw *(Harpagophytum procumbens):* pharmacological and clinical studies. *Ann Rheum Dis* 1981;40(6):632.
49. Pinget M, Lecomte A. The effects of Harpagophytum capsules (Arkocaps) in degenerative rheumatology. *Med Actuelle* 1985;12(4):65–67 [In French].
50. Dahout C. *J Pharm Belg* 1980;35(2):143–49.
51. Pickles H. *Devil's Claw: Its Remarkable Medicinal Properties* [a pamphlet], Reforma AG, Postfach, 6300 Zug Switzerland. [Citing: Yin Peida Yang Xiuyan. Preliminary clinical observation on treatment of 40 cases of arthritis with Pagosid. Branch of Rheumatology and Clinical Immunology, First Affiliated Hospital, Sun Yat Sen University of Medical Science; Wu Qifu, et al. Clinical effectiveness of Pagosid in treatment of arthritis. Department of Rheumatology, First Military Hospital, Nanfang Hospital; Cui Jinfang Shi Puzhen. Preliminary observation on treatment of arthritis with Pagosid. Department of Rheumatology, People's Hospital of Guandong Province.]

BIBLIOGRAPHY

The Arthritis Foundation. *Understanding Arthritis*. Edited by Irving Kushner, Ann Forer, and Ann McGuire. New York: Charles Scribner's Sons/ Macmillan, 1984.

Berkow, Robert and Anthony Fletcher, editors. *The Merck Manual*, 16th ed. Rahway, N.J.: M.B. Merck Research Laboratories, 1992.

Bradley, Peter, editor. *British Herbal Compendium*, vol. 1. Bournemouth, Dorset: British Herbal Medicine Association, 1992.

Brinker, Francis and Edward K. Alstat. *Eclectic Dispensary of Botanical Therapeutics*, vol. 2. Sandy, Ore.: Eclectic Medical Publications, 1995.

Brown, Donald, editor. *Quarterly Review of Natural Medicine 1994*. Seattle, Wash.: Natural Products Research Consultants, 1994.

Bruneton, Jean. *Pharmacognosy, Phytochemistry, Medicinal Plants*. Paris: Lavoisier Tec and Doc/Intercept Ltd., 1995.

Chang, H-M and P P-H But, editors. *Pharmacology and Applications of Chinese Materia Medica*, vol. 2. Translated by S C-S Yeung, L-L Wang, and Sih Cheng-Yao. Singapore: World Scientific Publishers, Toh Tuck Link, 1986. (http://www.worldscientific.com)

DeSmet, P.A.G.M., K. Keller, R. Hansel, and R. F. Chandler, editors. *Adverse Effects of Herbal Drugs*. New York: Springer Verlag, 1997.

BIBLIOGRAPHY

Duke, James. *CRC Handbook of Medicinal Herbs.* Boca Raton, Fl.: CRC Press, Inc., 1985.

Ebadi, Manuchair S. *CRC Desk Reference of Clinical Pharmacology (CRC Desk Reference Series).* Boca Raton, Fl.: CRC Press, Inc., 1997.

Evans, W.C. *Trease & Evans' Pharmacognosy,* 13th ed. Bailliére Tindall, 1989.

Hardin, Joseph G. and Gesina L. Longenecker. *Handbook of Drug Therapy in Rheumatic Disease: Pharmacology and Clinical Aspects.* New York: Little, Brown, 1992.

Horvilleur, Alain. *The Family Guide to Homeopathy.* Health and Homeopathy Publishing, Inc., 1986.

Jacob, Karen L., editor. *Why Arthritis?: Searching for the Cause and Cure of Rheumatoid Disease.* Preface by Harold W. Clark. Tampa Bay, Fl.: Axelrod Publishing, 1997.

Jones, Kenneth. *Cat's Claw: The Healing Vine of Peru.* Seattle, Wash.: Sylvan Press, 1995.

Leung, Albert, and Steven Foster. *Encyclopedia of Common Natural Ingredients Used in Foods, Drugs, and Cosmetics.* New York: John Wiley and Sons, Inc., 1996.

McGuffin, Michael, Christopher Hobbs, Roy Upton, and Alicia Goldberg, editors. *American Herbal Products Association's Botanical Safety Handbook.* Boca Raton, Fl.: CRC Press, Inc., 1997.

Mowrey, Daniel. *Herbal Tonic Therapies.* New Canaan, Conn.: Keats Publishing, 1993.

Murray, Michael. *The Healing Power of Herbs.* Rocklin, Calif.: Prima, 1995.

Murray, Michael and Joseph Pizzorno. *Encyclopedia of Natural Medicine.* Rocklin, Calif.: Prima, 1991.

Samuelsson, Gunnar. *Drugs of Natural Origin.* Stockholm: Swedish Pharmaceutical Press, 1992.

Saul, Sheldon. *The Doctor's Vitamin and Mineral Encyclopedia.* Simon and Schuster, 1990.

Scammell, Henry and Thomas McPherson Brown. *The Arthritis Breakthrough: The Road Back.* New York: M. Evans and Company, Inc., 1993.

Schwitters, Bert with Jacques Masquelier. *OPC in Practice.* Rome, Italy: Alfa Omega Editrice, 1993.

Sobel, Dava and Arthur C. Klein. *Arthritis: What Works.* New York: St. Martin's Press, 1989.

Tyler, Varro. *The Honest Herbal.* Binghamton, N.Y.: Pharmaceutical Products Press, 1993.

Utsinger, Peter D. and Nathan J. Zvaifler. *Rheumatoid Arthritis: Etiology, Diagnosis, Management.* Edited by George E. Ehrlich. New York: J.B. Lippincott, 1985.

Weiner, Michael with Janet Weiner. *Weiner's Herbal.* Mill Valley, Calif.: Quantum Books, 1990.

Weiss, Rudolf. *Herbal Medicine.* Beaconsfield, UK: Beaconsfield/Arcanum, 1988.

Werbach, Melvyn and Michael Murray. *Botanical Influences on Illness.* Tarzana, Calif.: Third Line Press, 1994.

Wichtl, Max. *Herbal Drugs and Phytopharmaceuticals.* Edited by Norman Bisset. Boca Raton, Fl.: Medpharm/CRC Press, 1994.

INDEX